INOCHI ENERGY MEDICINE

Any misspellings, misconceptions, or misinterpretations of individuals, terminologies, or systems are not intentional. I seek to convey, not confront or confuse. To quote Kahlil Gibran, *"Half of what I say is meaningless, but I say it so the other half may reach you."*

All proceeds support the work of IAALM, a 501(c)(3) health advancement organization established in 2002 to further the work and discoveries of Masahilo M. Nakazono, founder of Kototama Life Medicine.

INOCHI ENERGY MEDICINE
A Guide to Kototama Life Medicine

Teachings of Masahilo M. Nakazono Osensei
Studies by Thomas E. Duckworth,
Doctor of Kototama Life Medicine.

Thomas E. Duckworth

IAALM Press

©2018
©2023

INOCHI ENERGY MEDICINE
Diagnosis and Treatment
History, Evolution, and Findings –
A Journey

Veneration

Neem Karoli Baba Maharaj-ji

exemplifying the sacredness and power of spoken words and silence, leading to Masahilo M. Nakazono and the Kototama Principle.

In Honor and Celebration

Masahilo M. Nakazono

Founder – Teacher of Kototama Life Medicine

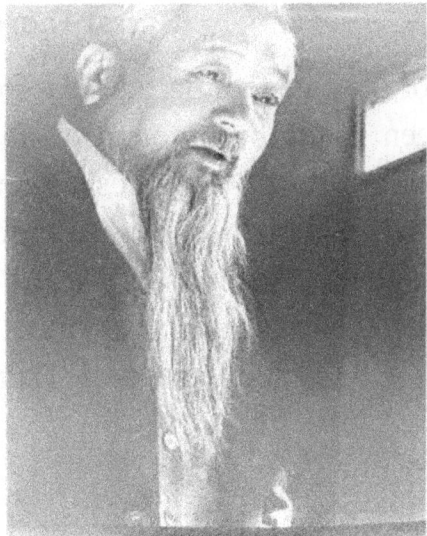

DEDICATION

to

Masahilo Nakazono Osensei, who always said,
"Know!"

Sharon Reed, who always says, "Yes!"

Gratitude

Sharon Reed

She teaches through unconditional love,
unlimited support, constant consideration, and
extraordinary wit. Thank you, Sharon.

Garret Thornburg

For the past four decades, Garrett Thornburg has
been in the background of all my professional
studies and activities with Masahilo M.
Nakazono Osensei. He has endorsed, encouraged,
inquired, questioned, and has continually
provided fantastic support. I have gratitude,
Garrett, just not the words. Thank you very much.

Acknowledgments

I am grateful to the many unnamed who have contributed toward completing this effort. You have not hesitated to endorse this mission to bring Masahilo M. Nakazono Osensei's teachings to the vanguard of natural medicine and consciousness expansion.

It is optimal, when journeying the inner landscape, to travel with those you love, and whenever I looked, there they were:

Ted Hall, DOM, L.Ac., my student and friend of many years, carries fire in his heart, humor in his voice, and an extraordinary commitment to Osensei's discoveries and passion.

Tracy Conrad, DOM, an immeasurable friend, in and out of the clinic, pays attention without seeking it and bubbles from within while attempting to satiate her thirst for knowledge. She has pursued Kototama Life Medicine with no plan except to eliminate feline allergies. Her relentless quest to learn the subtleties and brilliance of Japanese medicine has stimulated my studies. For her, I have much thankfulness and respect.

Jason R. Hackler, DOM, L.Ac., began his studies of Kototama Life Medicine in 1994; he has not stopped. He has made this his life's work, and we are all helped by his relentless dedication to healing. I have benefitted from his skill development for over a quarter of a century.

Thank you.

INOCHI ENERGY MEDICINE

Diagnosis and Treatment

History, Evolution, and Findings –

A Journey

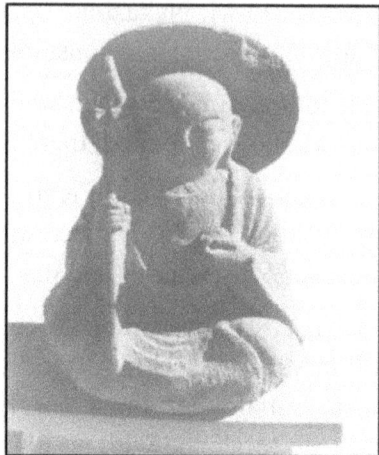

Jizo Bosatsu

Compassionate Buddha of ancestral wisdom

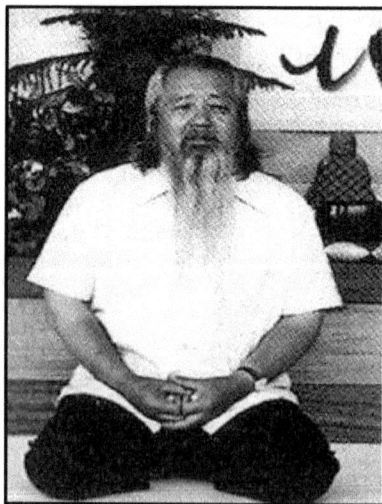

Masahilo. M. Nakazono

"There is one meridian, and its pulse is Chu Myaku."

"Anyone writing a creative work knows that you open, yield yourself, and the book talks to you and builds itself. To a certain extent, you become the carrier of something given to you from what has been called the Muses—or, in biblical language, 'God.' This is not fantasy; it is a fact. Since inspiration comes from the unconscious, and since the unconscious minds of the people of any small society have much in common, what the shaman or seer brings forth is waiting to be brought forth in everyone. So, when one hears the seer's story, one responds, 'Aha! This is my story. This is something that I had always wanted to say but wasn't able to say.' There has to be a dialogue, an interaction between the seer and the community."

Joseph Campbell (w/Bill Moyers), **The Power of Myth**

A Thought

Concerning studying and awakening the "energy body:" the current of the Universe manifesting in human life and consciousness, the vital life force, the gateway to (IE) dimension, the dimension of the soul that is the "soul" and its wisdom: Start with the reminder that what is sought will not be attained through seeking. To gain, let go.

"The way that can be spoken of is not the way.
The name that can be named is not the name.
The nameless is the beginning of the myriad forms.
The named is the mother of ten thousand things.
Therefore,
Those who seek the way without desire Will
sense it subtly.
Those with desire
Will see that which they seek and desire."

(Lao Tzu)

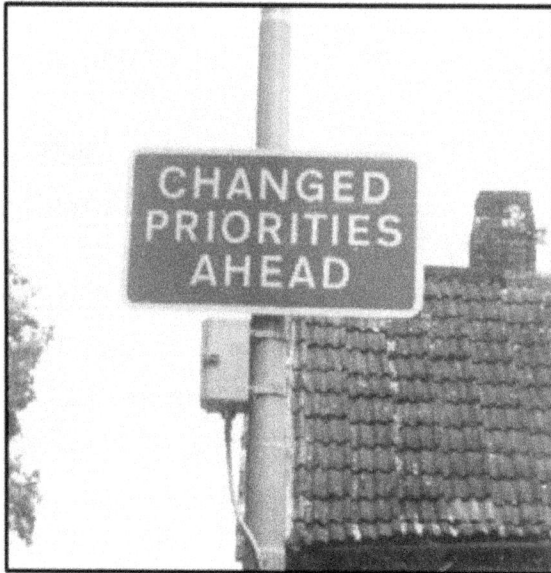

Road sign in England

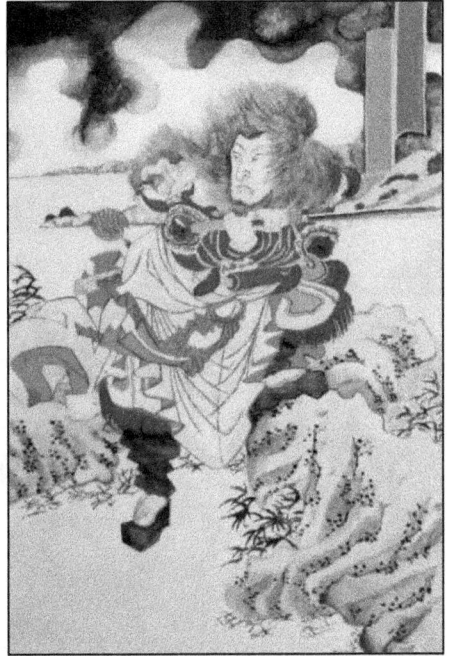

A postcard. Artist unknown (replicated by Judy Sawyer, Santa Fe, 1989)

"The Way is in the training.
Become acquainted with every (healing) art.
Know the ways of all professions.
Distinguish between gain and loss.
Develop intuitive judgment.
Perceive things that cannot be seen.
Pay attention to trifles.
Do nothing which is of no use."
Musashi Miyamoto
- Book of the Five Rings

Contents

CHAPTER ONE
PROLOGUE
1

CHAPTER TWO
ORIGINS
10

CHAPTER THREE
ENTER THE BARBARIA
36

CHAPTER FOUR
ETHOS
45

CHAPTER FIVE
KOTOTAMA PRINCIPLE
53

CHAPTER SIX
QI DEVELOPMENT
69

CHAPTER SEVEN
BREATHING
87

CHAPTER EIGHT
HAND SPIRIT QI TEATE
101

CHAPTER NINE
TEATE TREATMENT
WITH MOXIBUSTION AND HARI
140

CHAPTER TEN
KOTOTAMA INOCHI PULSE DIAGNOSIS
178

APPENDIX: OSENSEI'S 108 WARRIOR-PRIESTS
219

GLOSSARY
232

CHAPTER ONE
PROLOGUE

FINGER ON THE
PULSE

I handed him the film sheet, an x-ray of my left index finger. *"Come,"* he instructed, and we went outside, where he held the film up toward the sun and examined it. The x-ray showed an index finger that had been crushed and now hosted an antibiotic-resistant staphylococcus infection with gangrene. It was a digit the medical professionals said had to be amputated.

"Do you want your finger cut off?" asked the Japanese master. *"No, Sensei,"* I answered. He laughed. "I would not want my finger cut off either," he replied with more laughter. "Come back in." I followed him back into his clinic. It was the spring of 1973. I have been following him ever since. He made a few comments concerning the practice among pickpockets and common thieves in traditional Japan who would cut off the offender's index finger if they found one of them stealing from the group. That way, the hapless thief is forever branded as a petty thief of petty thieves. Sensei pondered aloud if it was more than a coincidence that I was losing my index finger. What karma had I created that led to this disaster? He was laughing the whole time he questioned my moral character.
"Albi," he finally advised,

"You must make albi for your finger."

Nobody knew about albi, this food medicine, or where to find it. My searches and inquiries brought me nothing.

The surgeons told me that if I did not have my finger amputated soon, I would lose my whole hand. I returned to Sensei's office: "Sensei, I cannot find albi."

"I did not say to get albi; I said to get taro root and make albi," he answered. "I said taro, taro!" Me: "I'm sorry, Sensei. How do you spell that?"

I was learning. I learned that albi consists of taro root, ginger root, flour, and enough water to form a putty-like paste. I learned that an albi plaster is one of the most potent extracting agents for removing foreign objects from the body. I have employed it to remove splinters from children, shrapnel from war veterans, cancer from patients, staph, gangrene, and bone chips from my finger. I have successfully used it to address traumatic pain, arthritic swelling, fractured bones, dislocated joints, headache, blunt trauma injury, and fever.

It took time, but I obtained raw taro root in Chinatown, New York City through friends. Now, one can buy it on the Internet already dried and powdered, with ginger added.

That was my first direct interaction with Masahilo M. Nakazono. Previously I had witnessed the results of his treatment skills on my domestic partner's Ménierè's Syndrome. His unique meridian therapy skills provided twice a week for many months, along with a natural, grain- based diet with phases of active dietary detoxification, brought about a cure for what medical doctors had deemed incurable. His treatment of my son's outbreak of warts:

eliminate sugar and red meat, rub warts with raw eggplant. That eliminated warts quickly. In addition, his burdock root remedy saved my daughter from an unnecessary appendectomy.

These I witnessed, but I was slow to seek his care when I had my infected finger to deal with, even though my partner strongly urged me to consult him. I was exploring alternatives to everything at that time in my life, but for my finger, I knew I needed *"Western medicine."* I even said, *"I need a real doctor."* I was wrong on so many levels. I was being led to a "real doctor."

A worsening condition and an insistent mate caused me to act. I finally presented myself to Dr. Masahilo M. Nakazono, teacher and healer extraordinaire. I arrived with my xray and left with confidence my finger was savable.

The journey with my finger lasted months. I searched for taro root, found, and acquired taro, made albi plaster, and changed the bandaged plaster every eight hours. I continued with the plaster constantly for over two months. It completely healed my finger. I received a couple of treatments during that period while Sensei monitored my care of the finger. He reinforced the confidence I had in what was happening. We spoke extraordinarily little; each session was less than thirty minutes. Sensei scheduled his patients every thirty minutes. He was never late for his next patient. Thus, my second extended communication with Sensei occurred some months later. My finger had healed entirely. I had no issues that required Sensei's attention. I lived over an hour's drive from Santa Fe, and I had much work to do on my homestead now that I had the use of my left hand again. However, I wanted to thank him and express my gratitude for his life-altering medicine's effects on my family and me. So, I made an appointment to see him at the end of his workday. Again, to say thank you.

"Just a few minutes, please."

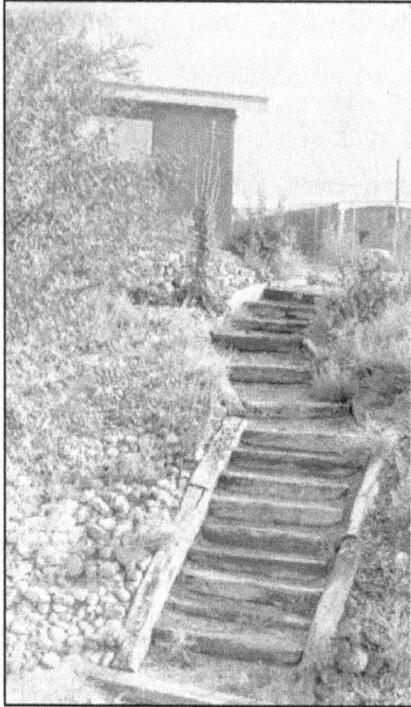

Steps from the parking lot to the dojo.

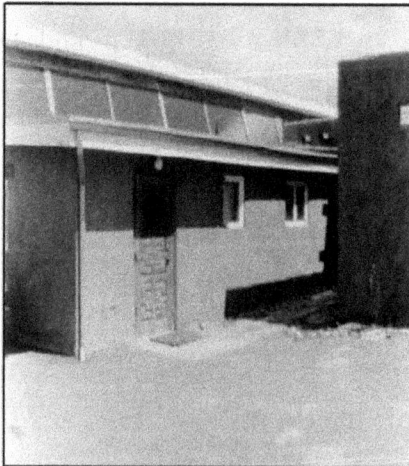

The public entrance to the dojo.

He met me in his dojo, recently built onto his clinic, where he conducted classes concerning the study and practice of the Kototama Principle, shared veneration of Jizo Bosatsu, taught aikido, and offered natural medicine talks. The building blended a Shinto-Buddhist temple and martial arts school constructed in Southwest architectural "pueblo" style and made of adobe. It was secure and peaceful.

We sat in quiet for a moment. *"Why do you wish to talk to me?"* asked Sensei. I had a vague idea of what I would say, not the exact words. I did not have a prepared speech; just wanted to express my appreciation humbly and gratefully. I wanted to say "thank you" for saving my finger.

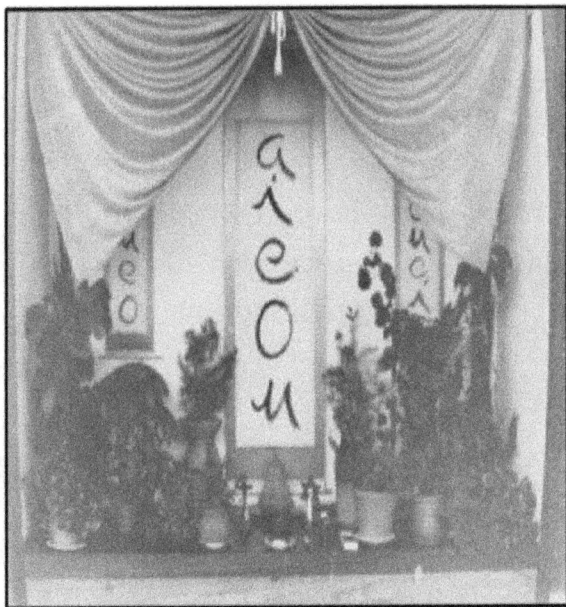

Shomen– Jizo Bosatsu Shrine

"Sensei," I could hear the words coming out of my mouth; they were not forming in my brain; they were coming out of my mouth. I was experiencing my thoughts, hearing my thoughts, as I was speaking, hearing my words at the same time Sensei was hearing them. "Sensei, I need to know what you know," I blurted out.

I was seeing, hearing, and feeling my mind express my heart. I did not know what I needed to know, but I was sure I NEEDED to know what he knew. He was a traditional healer of body, mind, and spirit. I should walk close to him.

Sensei Nakazono looked at me for a brief period, ten microseconds, ten minutes, ten days; who knows?

"Yes, you do," he responded. "You start with the Kototama sounds."

Quickly I responded, "Sensei, I have read all your published lectures and both of your books, *The Messiah's Return* and *Kototama,*[*] and I don't understand anything I have read."

With seriousness, mirth, teacher authority, and elder brother love, Nakazono replied, "You cannot get the Kototama Principle by reading, only by doing

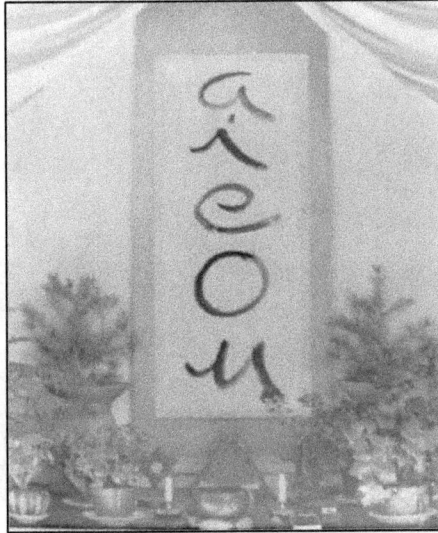

Kototama Futonorito Order of Mother Sounds,
Nakazono Osensei's "alter" - Kototama Institute

*Osensei's books are available at www.Kototamabooks.com.
Additional recipes: **Natural Medicine from the Kitchen**,
eBook, & paperback www.amazon.com.

THE DOJO ALIVE

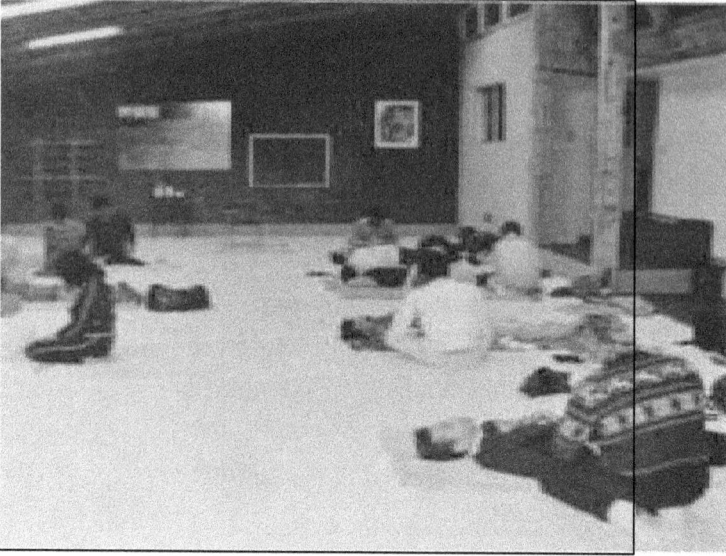

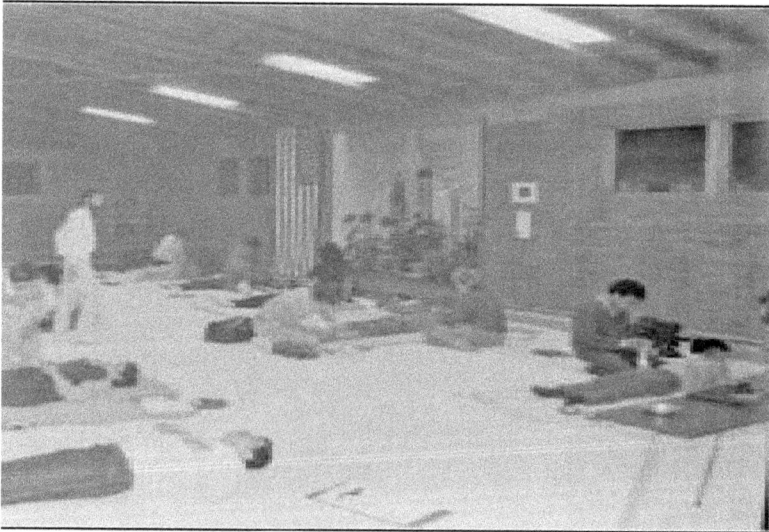

Clinical Studies

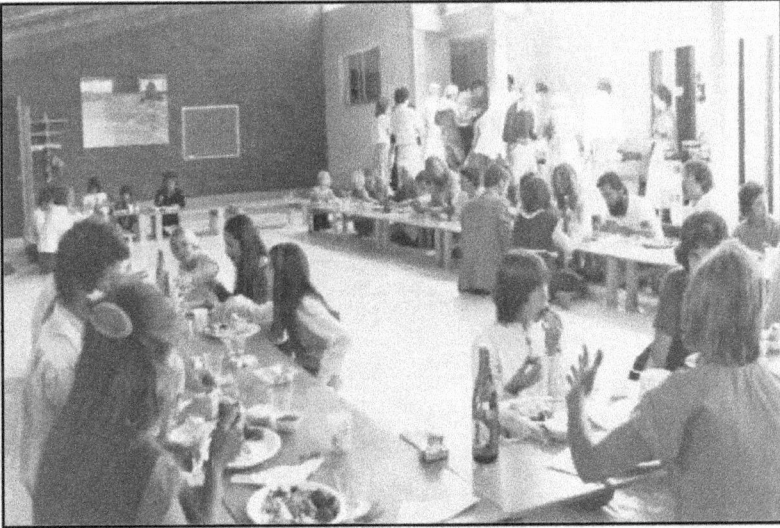

Kototama Institute Family Meal

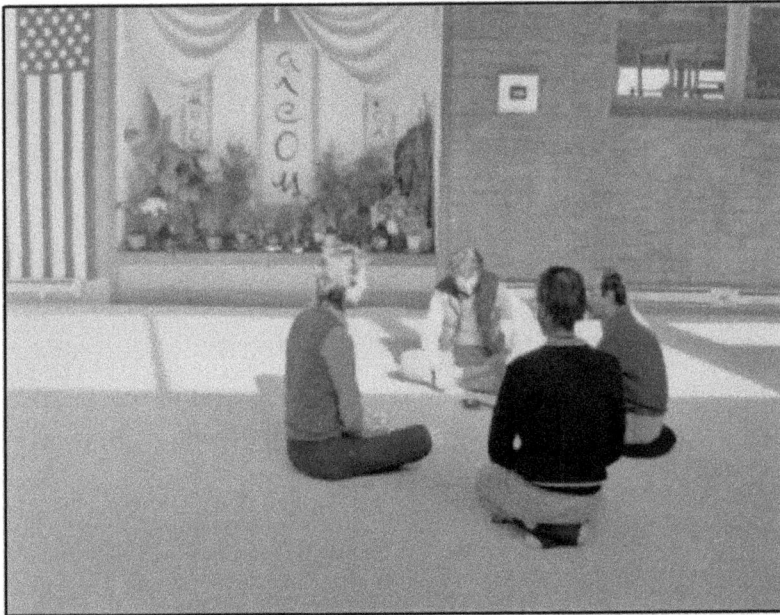

Senior Students

CHAPTER TWO

ORIGINS

When I encountered Nakazono's medicine, I could not spell the word acupuncture. It was 1972. All my experiences of Asian healing arts, Shinto rituals, Japanese Buddhist practices, and Japanese martial arts came to me through the gift of my teacher. All my studies occurred under Masahilo M. Nakazono, Osensei, from 1973 through 1988.

Healthcare has long been a cultural practice in many societies, including East Asia and the Middle East, the Indigenous people of the Americas, and the traditional practitioners of Europe and the Nordic regions; some have health systems thousands of years old. The oldest systems in continuous practice originated in India, Persia, and China. My studies and practices are in Japanese traditional medicine and Hindu spiritual and health sciences. It is from the "East" that we have come to understand the link between spirituality and natural science. Thus, while the concept of the human as a holistic body/mind/spirit actuality is new to the western world, yogis, physicians, philosophers, and farmers of East Asia have thrived for thousands of years with this knowledge and understanding.

The principle of treating body energy channels, meridians, was set down in *Nanjing*[1], a 2,500-year-old healing arts text. This science has been studied and utilized continuously. Our medicine is 2,500 years long its way. It is a 2,500-year-long book still being written. We are an aspect of that way. There are a lot of blank spaces on these pages that we each must fill, so the next generation has a gift equal to the one we have.

The masters, through the ages, have provided various explanations of the Nanjing and the other canon of traditional Chinese medicine, Neijing, and have taught multiple ways and descriptions of the pulses. These interpretations are presented in symbols and metaphors, reflections in the mirror of self-awareness, thus, misidentified as reality.

The study and understanding of acupuncture evolved within the cultural, linguistic, social, and ecological environment in which it is practiced. Consequently, there are distinct distinctions between

---

[1] **Nanjing - The Classic of Difficult Issues,** compiled around the first to second century, addresses issues relevant to the information in the Neijing, the canon of internal medicine also termed the **Yellow Emperor's Classic of Internal Medicine**, compiled 500 years earlier. Nanjing presents the wrist pulses diagnosis.

"Chinese" and "Japanese" acupuncture and an evolving North American acupuncture.

Furthermore, within this new evolving paradigm, the influences of the "classics" will differ as they are restudied and applied anew. Consequently, the definition of the classics may be redefined.

There are various "schools" of traditional Asian medicine. There are differing views of the actions and functions, and even the existence of the anatomical conduits termed meridians (more accurately called myaku, space/channel/vein of pulsatory motion). There are different values of the four aspects of diagnosis, differing interpretations of pulse diagnosis, the significance given to the body/mind/spirit phenomenon, and the sense and sensibilities concerning the classics. There are libraries full of diagnosis studies, including pulse diagnosis interpretations and significances. Traditional and contemporary encyclopedias cover the causes of hundreds of diseases. I seek to provide a means by which one may grasp the path of Masahilo M. Nakazono. So that we might understand; as Wang Shu-he, director of the Imperial Medical Academy during the Jin Dynasty, said in The Pulse Classic; the "far-reaching imports" and "enigmatic" arcane transmissions and interpretations of the old classics.

The Five Element theory that classifies all things as wood, fire, water, metal, and earth still generates discussion and debate; it is a theory, not a law. The original writings concerning traditional oriental medicine, being cryptic and of an ancient tongue, have had various interpretations and applications throughout the past twenty-five centuries. The evolutionary journey of interpreting Go Gyo, the Five Element theory, took yet another turn when the pattern became redefined by Masahilo M. Nakazono.

This is a presentation of my studies and practice of Kototama Natural Life Therapy Inochi Medicine for your further studies, a clinical workbook for the serious student of Inochi Life. I welcome this opportunity to share a unique expression of meridian therapy.

KOTOTAMA LIFE MEDICINE

Kototama Life Medicine focuses on the diagnosis of seventeen pulses and the provision of Kototama Meridian Therapy. Kototama Life Medicine evolved through the studies of the Kototama Principle within the traditional systems of classic Five Element meridian therapy, traditional oriental medicine, and Japanese naturopathic medicine.

Independent of his clinical work, Masahilo M. Nakazono Osensei spent decades studying the Kototama Principle, In studying the Kojiki and the Takenouchi Documents, ancient religious texts, he realized new light was being shed on ancient understandings of the principle of Life Energy (Qi), the meaning of meridian, and the more profound implications of the Five Element concept.

Osensei had been studying Qi through martial arts for over a half-century and through meridian therapy for over 30 years. He knew of the concept of Life Energy manifesting from apriori[2] (before form) to aposteriori[3] (form) and returning to apriori (formless).   This has been addressed by many spiritual and philosophical teachers, hermits, wandering warriors, gurus, yogis, lunatics, and psychedelic journeyers.

---

[2] "From the earlier." In the context of Kototama studies, apriori is what exists before form, the infinite.

[3] "From the later." In the context of Kototama studies, aposteriori is what exists in form. The actual expression of the sounds gives them form, which defines them as aposteriori, the finite

It is the focal point of all journeyers, whether they know it or not.

As his awareness in Kototama deepened, Osensei more clearly recognized our conscious involvement in Life's formation, maintenance, and evolution. Life itself is the propelling force, the only force. Life and the Universe are one. Life is a noun; Universe is a verb.

"The voice (Kototama) is the self-expression of Life (Inochi)."
Ogasawara Koji Sensei

He studied and practiced until his studies of the Kototama Principle brought him to where he could stand in the tangible world and grasp the cosmic dance of the chaotic world, witnessing life coming into being and expressing the energy of life. He found all this in the pulses.

After ten years of studies with Ogasawara Sensei and applying the Kototama Principle, Osensei grasped the connection between the Five Element theory, wood/fire/earth/metal/water, and the five "mother sounds," A/I/U/E/O. He realized the classic Five Element paradigm aligns with the Kanagi order of sound manifesting consciousness, one of the three orders of consciousness in the studies of the Kototama Principle. He and every other practitioner of Five Element meridian therapy diagnosed and treated according to reasoning within the Kanagi (A/I/U/E/O) order of consciousness. The Kanagi order worked with a treatment success rate of about 70 percent. Practitioners with higher success rates seemed to use intuition and hyo-ji (treating symptoms) in addition to the Five Element principles. He began clinically researching the treatment efficacy of utilizing the Sugaso (A/O/U/E/I) and the Futonorito (A/I/E/O/U) orders in the Five Element paradigm. He found that treating according to the Kanagi order (current Five Element paradigm) was more effective than the Sugaso order. Treating in the Futonorito order increased his success rate to over 90 percent. His research and discoveries radically changed his perspective and altered his diagnostic viewpoint and treatment protocols. It guided him to reconsider his usage of needling (hari), moxibustion (kyu), and tactile (teate) treatments, and they changed accordingly.

This lineage, the Kototama Way of Pulse and Meridian Therapy, includes the twelve pulses in the three wrist positions - traditionally termed Ryokubu-jio and "both hands, six pulses," utilizing sunko-kanjo-shaku-chu pulse (sun, kan, shaku positions) - and includes Chu Myaku (middle pulse, Life Pulse, stomach pulse) and <u>Jingei myaku, the pulse at Jingei[4], </u> lower Yo Mei (stomach) #9 and their collective analysis.

In addition to the methods of classical acupuncture and moxibustion, Osensei unified Five Element shiatsu, anma[5,] and ampuku[6], Sakai Hon Rei Teate (the unique abdominal laying on of hands taught by Buddhist monk Sakai Sensei), and restoration therapy in the establishment of Kototama Meridian Therapy and his treatment protocols.

---

[4] Jingei - Pulse diagnosis that compares the carotid pulse at lower Yo Mei (St) #9 with the radial pulse at upper Tai Yin (lung or Lu) #9 (taien), sun position. Nakazono Osensei was protective of his new understanding of the Go Gyo ("Five Elements") achieved through his twenty-year journey that included the most in-depth studies of the Kototama Principle. The revelation of the jingei diagnosis demonstrates the harmonization of the Futonorito Five Element paradigm.

5. Anma - "Push-Pull" traditional Japanese massage. Stretching, rotating, squeezing, pressure, rubbing, and kneading to stimulate vital energy. The functional reliability of physical systems is sedated with pressure (an) and normalized by rubbing (ma). The practice uses the palm, fingers, and thumb to stimulate blood circulation, releasing stagnated blood in skin and muscle and addressing all circulatory congestion, tension, and stiffness. Historically, treatment occurred on the floor to enhance therapeutics. The modern method, on a table, provides more relaxation.

6 Ampuku - Abdominal massage developed as a profession in Japan several hundred years ago. It was followed by fukushin, combining abdominal diagnosis and kampo (herbal) treatment. Kampo, Japanese herbal medicine, was refined in the seventeenth century by Yoshimasu Todo, who developed a refined technique of abdominal palpation, fukushin, to provide additional information in determining the appropriate herbal formula.

Furthermore, he uncovered its association with tai kyoku (tai chi), yin/yang, pulse diagnosis, and the source and purpose of human Life Energy and its soul. Through his work, we have Kototama Life Medicine, a system of energy therapy grounded in an Five Element relationship with the five mother sounds and a therapeutic system of sound meditation and medicinal application involving Qi Gong practice, breath work, handwork, movement, acupuncture, moxibustion, dietary practices, folk, and herbal medicine, shonishin, kappo [7], and sotai [8], as well as traditional and contemporary methods of acute care— all tied to social responsibility.

Through his applied studies of the Kototama Principle and focused attention to pulse diagnosis and the connection between jingei pulse diagnosis and the principle of San Yin/San Yo, Osensei utilized all his varied healing techniques to formulate an integrated system of meridian therapy. Furthermore, his bodywork techniques progressed through his studies and dedication to the principle that a person who maintains balanced meridians is in the most optimal position to live a whole and healthy life. He ceased referring to his work as acupuncture or Japanese medicine. Instead, Osensei named his healing art form, Kototama Life (Inochi) Medicine, or, alternatively, Natural Life Therapy.

Kototama Life Medicine is the guidance of universal energy, Qi, manifesting in human form and expanding human consciousness. This universal energy creates the meridians and the human vowel sounds: (A I E O U). This Qi is expressed through Life-Spirit (A), Life-Will (I), Life-Force (E), Life-Mind (O), and Life-Form (U).

---

[7] Kappo – "Resuscitation Method"/ "Restoration Therapy" healing techniques for physical body repair. This includes tsubo treatment, tactile stimulation, physical manipulation, and alignment techniques.

[8] Sotai – A system of simple movements devised by Keizo Hashimoto, MD, to restore and maintain balanced posture and movement.

KOTOTAMA INSTITUTE

Nakazono Osensei opened the Kototama Institute in 1977, providing seminars and workshops. In September 1978, he initiated a two-year training program in oriental medicine and acupuncture and aimed to train one hundred individuals in Kototama Life Medicine. Two years later, it became a threeyear program.

Sharing his wealth as an expression of gratitude to his newfound home, America. His wealth consisted of fifty-plus years of discipline and proficiency in kendo, karate, judo, and aikido; his practice of Buddhist and Shinto principles coupled with fortyplus years of practice and understanding of traditional Japanese natural medicine, all integrated through the Kototama Principle.

The purpose of this holistic, transdisciplinary, multifaceted reinterpretation of Five Element meridian therapy is to:

1. Grasp *"who is I am"* and heal self,
2. Grasp the pulses and heal 'other,'
3. Grasp the Kototama Principle and heal society.

He provided a strict, disciplined training program. He expected his students to conduct themselves as students with all the humbleness, quietude, and gratefulness of any young, ignorant student. His students were all ages; most of his early natural medicine students were in their thirties.

"Three types of students will come to study Natural Life Therapy at the Institute:

*Those who cannot stand to see the suffering of humanity, whether physically or spiritually.

**Those who are very seriously searching to see the innermost mechanisms of the universe.

***Those interested in creating a professional life for themselves in society.

Only the first two types of students will be accepted.

The student who is interested in making either a name or money by using acupuncture has no capacity to heal, and instead of helping society, would become another harmful element. The Kototama Institute has no desire to train this type of person."

Brochure Announcing the School of Natural Life Medicine

He had no time or tolerance for adults with heads full of themselves. He would advise them to go and start their own schools because they knew so much and did not need to be a student any longer. He attempted to guide rude, self-serving, egotistical adults to be considerate of others and to be part of the healing instead of the injuring. The minute a class began, and the dojo (school) door closed, anyone not in their place was excluded from classes and clinical practice that day. He considered being late rude; he did not support rudeness in a healing environment.

He tried to protect all his students from being distracted in their studies; he wanted to protect us from distracting each other. Ego and (O) dimension (habitual thinking) bounced everywhere. Students were not to share notes without Sensei's permission. It was too easy for a student to misunderstand and cause misinformation. It was better to keep misunderstanding of phenomena to oneself. Pulses daily, the practice of meridian treatment procedures based on the pulses daily, compare pulse diagnosis and abdominal diagnosis to grasp the connections and the various levels of diagnostic information provided by those sources, compare and analyze the range and limitations of these diagnostic and treatment approaches. We treated only fellow students under his direct supervision for over a year before being allowed to practice on anyone else, even a family member.

All our studies focused on Qi; all our studies focused on the pulses. The studies began with "Hand QI Exercise," a union of mindbody-spirit through focused attention to breathing and Qi as exemplified in the discoveries of Ueshiba Osensei, founder of aikido; the teachings of Sakai Sensei and the work of Nakazono Osensei.

We treated each other with teate, moxibustion, natural diet, and Kototama sound for over a year before being shown and allowed to practice "the way of the needle." Sensei taught his students to treat the meridians with the hands, and only then taught how to use needles as an extension of oneself. This is how he practiced; this is how he taught. The treatment is in the diagnosis, the diagnosis is in the pulses, and the treatment is in the hands.

He was strict because he was responsible for transmitting 2,500 years of studies and practice of one of the subtlest forms of the science of energy known to humankind to a handful of Westerners who knew nothing. His most challenging work was with those who thought they knew something.

Osensei taught us to correct all pulse imbalances with our handwork. Through the breath of both the patient and the practitioner, through an understanding of hands expressing tanden (the physical as well as Life Energy center), we were guided in providing ho (enhance) and sha (liberate). It also brought a method of meditation and centering in delivery of acupuncture, moxibustion one's spiritual journey, as well as the spiritual discipline necessary for the adequate delivery of acupuncture, moxibustion, and tactile therapy. He guided us in pain-free needling. First, we practiced individually, planting the needle into an orange, then we practiced planting the needle into an apple floating in a bowl of water. Each student had to present themselves to Sensei and demonstrate the ability to plant a needle in an apple bobbing in a bowl full of water without spilling a drop. The vessel was full to the brim, and if one drop of water fell from the container, the student failed and had to return, after additional practice, for another demonstration. Success meant we could now practice needling our thighs repeatedly until we could consistently apply the needling technique without bleeding, bruising, or discomfort. He taught nontraumatic direct moxa usage. We practiced on each other for many hours, developing gentleness and finesse. He guided us toward attentiveness and quick action for the sake of the patient. He was, as a teacher, a taskmaster; as a physician, a gentle warrior.

When Osensei opened his school, there was no adequate text to recommend to a student. The first textbooks on Chinese medicine I read were publications from China circa 1970. These textbooks provided Communist propaganda, seeking to equate dialectic materialism with the principle of yin/yang.

They were early examples of the technocratic movement toward the mechanical treatment of symptoms by blending traditional medicine, political philosophy, and biomedical practices with the current social paradigm of conflict and dominance.

Sensei would eventually write and publish *Law and Therapy of Natural Medicine*[9] in 1978.

Still, in these early days, there were no texts in English from Japan on meridians, tsubo (acupuncture point) location, usage, or contraindications, nor any historical or clinical experiences, except *Illustration of Acupuncture Points* (1977), self-described as "basic information concerning the location of the acupoint," published by Ido-No-NipponSha. It was my first commercially published meridian textbook.

---

9 Written and self-published for his students, the 1978 and 1979 editions were called the "Red Book" for the color of their covers. The 1980-81 edition was referred to as the "Gold Book" for the same reason; plus, it is quite rich.in information.

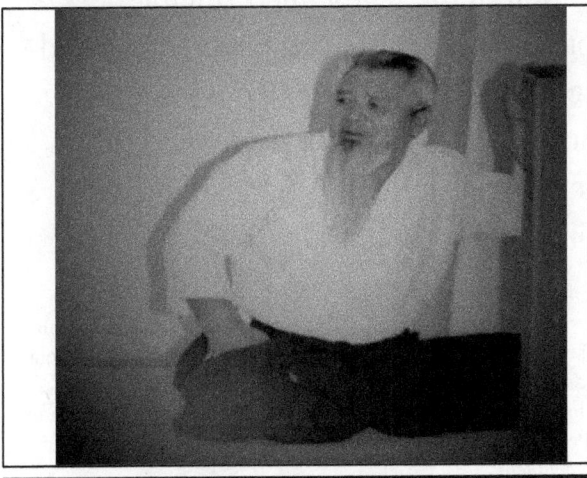

His son read tsubo location and usage notes from his Japanese acupuncture college studies, translating to English as he read. Sensei lectured day after day. As students, we frantically wrote with paper and pen, asked questions, and wrote more. We each had a copy of *Illustration of Acupuncture Points* and copious handwritten notes (including clinic notes from diagnosing and treating each other two to three times a week) for studying. At the end of the first year of studies, I had three large binders full of handwritten class and clinic notes. He spoke and demonstrated; I wrote and drew diagrams and body outlines with x's and arrows. His teaching and guidance were always within the framework of Kototama Life Energy and centered physically in the pulses. At the nouchi Documents.end of the second year, I had seven binders. Forty-one years later, I am still referencing the fifty-two binders of Sensei's information and teachings. He left so much of himself in his attempt to heal. Everything I do, or practice, is 'Nakazono's Way.'

'Nakazono's Way,' the therapeutics I have studied and practiced for more than forty years, is classic Five Element meridian therapy and pulse diagnosis, redefined and refined through the spiritual and clinical application of the Kototama Principle,[10] Kototama Life Medicine, or Natural Life Therapy, perceived and applied, by Osensei after he settled in New Mexico, established a revolutionary reinterpretation of Go Gyo (Five Elements), a fuller understanding of being human and our spiritual, mental, and physical place in the Universe.

---

10. Soul/Spirit/Power within the spoken sounds of human language wherein reality is created, and consciousness expressed. Nakazono Osensei was introduced to the sound principle through translations of the *Kojiki* and Takenouchi Documents during his studies under Ueshiba Osensei, founder of Aikido. His pursuit of understanding led him to Ogasawara Sensei, whose linage of Kototama studies trace to the nineteenth century Meiji Restoration Period and the family of calligraphers enlisted to translate the ancient scrolls known as the *Takenouchi Document*.

scrolls
known as the
*Takenouchi
Document*

Call it American acupuncture. I do.

Masahilo M. Nakazono Osensei strongly urged his students to study the way of pulses humbly. "In Japan," he repeatedly reminded us, "it is said that when you have taken the pulses of ten people every day for ten years, you may earn the title of Beginner."

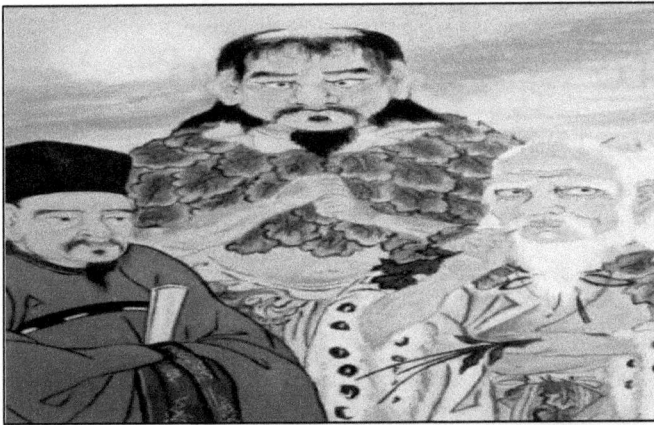

MASTERS
Legendary "Emperors," founders of the healing arts.
Recreated by Judy Sawyer, Santa Fe 1988,
from a black & white print of a Japanese scroll by Seibi Wake, 1798

Fu Hsi [2852-2738 BCE] - Father of the philosophy of tai chi and yin/yang and author of the *I Ching*; the inventor of writing, fishing with nets, and trapping and divination.

Shennong [2695 BCE], "Emperor of the Five Grains," the Divine Husbandman, and author of the *Divine Husbandman's Materia Medica.* He is considered the father of Chinese medicine and agriculture. He taught planting and harvesting, identified medicinal herbs, invented the plow, tamed the cow, yoked the horse, and cleared farmland with fire.

Huang-Ti [2697-2597 BCE] Mytho-historical ruler, traditionally credited with various innovations, from the Chinese calendar to sports. He wrote the *Yellow Emperor's Canon of Internal Medicine.*

"The human capacity is physical and spiritual. This world teaches us to manifest our physical abilities, but we must develop our spiritual capacity if we are to heal; if we are to be complete."
Nakazono Osensei, class notes, 1978

MASAHILO   NAKAZONO
May 22, 1918 October 8, 1994

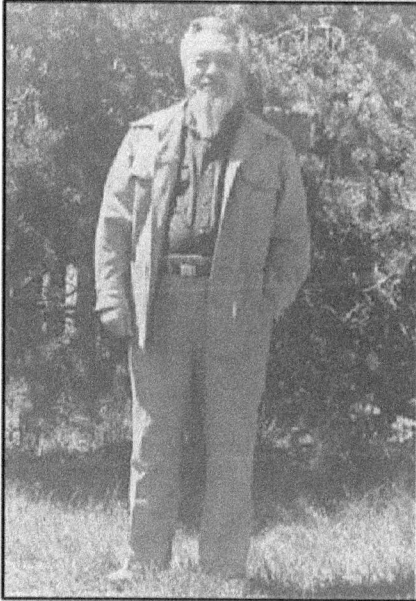

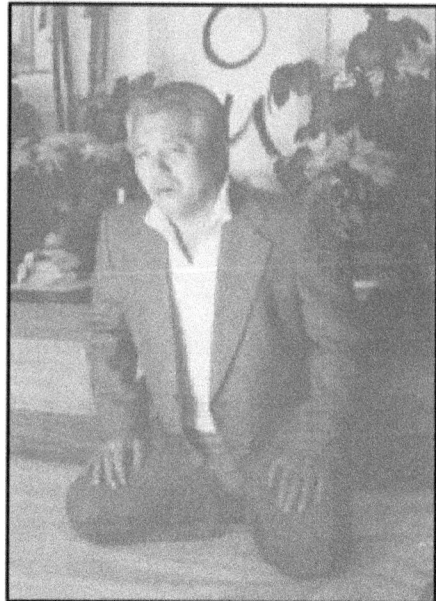

Osensei, Jizo Bosatsu Talk, 1985

Born May 22, 1918, in the southern Kagoshima Prefecture of Japan, Masahilo M. Nakazono was the son of a rice farmer and compulsive gambler who traveled throughout Japan and China in search of the big win. According to Osensei, his father inadvertently poisoned himself by habitually coloring his hair with coal oil. He died while on one of his trips to China. His mother, Chie Fuchigami-Nakazono, raised Masahilo and his two brothers, supplementing her rice field rental income as a nurse, midwife, and herbalist using foods, herbs, poultices, and massage. She was highly respected and widely recognized for her ability to turn breech babies. Demand for her services continued throughout Osensei's childhood, and he grew up helping her and learning traditional folk medicine.

Martial arts were also in his family tree. His great-grandfather, Kosuzume, was a sumo champion, and his uncle began teaching him the way of kendo when he was six; he ranked seventh dan when he retired. In school, he ran field and track. At age 12, he began the study of judo and continued until he achieved the rank of seventh dan. He became a judo champion by the age of 18 and completed kappo certification at 19. That same year, he began training in karate, achieving fifth dan. He was a direct student of Morihei Ueshiba Osensei, founder of Aikido. Under Ueshiba's guidance, Masahilo M. Nakazono founded the first aikido dojo outside of Japan in Singapore and was one of the early Japanese masters to introduce aikido in Europe.

While in Europe, he began his Kototama studies with Ogasawara Sensei. In the 1970s, he declined the rank of eighth dan from the World Aikido Federation. Ten years later, he retired from Aikido and all martial arts. He dedicated the last twenty years of his life to healing arts and spiritual practices. He departed France in 1972 and relocated to Santa Fe, New Mexico.

His formal training in Japanese medicine began in 1934 when he apprenticed with Dr. Juzo Motoyama, with whom he studied for the next six years. The Japanese army drafted him and sidetracked his studies for a few years. His tour with the Japanese army severely compromised his health. He contracted malaria, hepatitis, and parasites and was malnourished with an enlarged spleen and liver. The Australian doctors who mustered him out of the Japanese army told him he had six months to live. That spurred him to plunge deeper into the study and utilization of many healing forms. He discovered Oshawa Sensei while struggling with his health issues. His young wife, Harue Nakazono, also would not accept that prognosis. She began macrobiotic cooking for her husband and their two children. Madame Nakazono learned of Sakai Sensei and insisted her husband put himself under his care.

In the late '40s and early '50s, he was close to George Sakurazawa (a.k.a. George Oshawa), founder of the macrobiotic method of dietary healing. Oshawa sent Nakazono to Madras, India, to direct a macrobiotic hospital treating lepers and people with mental health conditions. They were treated with meals based on macrobiotic principles and individually prepared by Nakazono. It was there that Nakazono discovered a fundamental flaw in macrobiotic thinking: the idea that one diet fits all persons and conditions. Nakazono devised five basic diets he shared with Oshawa Sensei, who acknowledged him with a seventh-dan ranking in Macrobiotics and then dismissed him from further studies. Soon after, Oshawa announced that there would be seven elemental diets in macrobiotics.

In this same period, he was studying a new martial art form, aikido, with its founder, Morihei Ueshiba, who introduced him to the power of Kototama sound and the spiritual aspects of physical being.

In 1950, he turned thirty-two. Growth was taking place, and he began studying Shugendo Healing under Master Sakai, a Shugendo Buddhist monk. Sakai also introduced Nakazono to the veneration of Jizo Bosatsu, the bodhisattva of universal unity, protector of those lost in and through death. These studies included hands-on spiritual healing, which Nakazono Osensei termed Sakai Hon Rei Teate.

By 1958, he was in Vietnam, teaching judo and aikido to the South Vietnamese army as a combat technique instructor. Then, realizing that Vietnam was in a civil war with too much international manipulation, he resigned and, in 1961, relocated to France as an official representative of Aikikai Hombu, the original school of Aikido, through the International Aikido Federation. Over the next eleven years, he influenced thousands of students in Europe and North Africa before moving to the United States. It was in this era that he began Kototama studies with Ogasawara Sensei.

Initially, he studied the Kototama Principle as a 'spiritual exercise' independent of his clinical work and Aikido. However, as he experienced new light being shed on ancient understandings of the principle of Life Energy (Qi), his spiritual practices changed, as did his medicine. Furthermore, as he applied the Kototama Principle to the Five Element (Go Gyo) theory, he discovered a new relationship within the energetic flow of meridians, and a different interpretation of Go Gyo emerged.

By 1977, Masahilo M. Nakazono Osensei had established and begun teaching, Kototama teate, a merging of spiritual handwork, martial arts, traditional healing art, and Kototama sound meditation guided through Kototama diagnosis, particularly pulse and abdominal diagnosis.

In 1978, Osensei opened his school, the Kototama Institute, where the practice of aikido was, at first, a part of the curriculum. After that, however, he discontinued it because it promoted a sense of achievement and not the spirit of service; it philosophically advocates peace but does not promote healing.

He opened the Kototama Institute with the expressed purpose of sharing his wealth with his fellow citizens. His wealth included over a halfcentury of discipline and understanding of aikido, judo, karate, and kendo; his life- long practice of Buddhist and Shinto principles; forty years of study and knowledge of traditional Japanese natural medicine, especially pulse diagnosis, acupuncture, moxibustion, diet, and teate; and his study and understanding of the Kototama Principle. This holistic, transdisciplinary multi-faceted reinterpretation of diagnostic and treatment protocol of Five Element therapy he termed Kototama Life Medicine.

He wished to plant seeds for future growth.

The old Japanese system of keeping

"secrets" within a family was not only passé and counter-revolutionary but counter to his desire to live within a civilization that honors a total commitment to the life-being and empowerment of every individual. There are no secrets to keep; there are empowerments to share. There is no more time for separation; now is the time for unity. He stated his intent to pass his basic knowledge on to one hundred students. Within those hundred, he imagined encountering ten "doctoral students" with the desire to complete his Do, the way of Kototama Life Medicine.

The focus of these studies is to comprehend *"Who is I am,"* to heal the whole self, to understand the pulses to treat "other," and to comprehend the Kototama Principle to heal society. He believed we have the potential to develop conscious inter-expression of our equitable physical- mentalspiritual being. He sought to contribute to our collective destiny as practitioners, which he perceived to be our leadership in guiding the world from what he termed "the materialistic/scientific civilization" to a civilization wherein the sages act in harmonious regard for the mind/body/spirit of the citizenry - the entire species in its environment. Nakazono Osensei was "old school." When he said *"yes"* to a student applicant, he entered a contract to provide that student the state-of-the-art traditional training, to teach by feeding his heart to the student, serving it on a sword. He was saying "yes" to the principle that a teacher gives all of their self so that the next generation will have not only the ancient knowledge but the ancient spirit to the perseverance of the ancient knowledge, the ancient spirit, dedication, and capacity to be a steward of an unbroken lineage of clinical experience and skills that extend thousands of years and can only continue through this personal responsibility.

In addition to the pulses, Masahilo M. Nakazono Osensei thoroughly examined the patient's forms, signs, and expressed elements. To establish a diagnosis, he studied every facet and factor (listening, looking, questioning, touching). His understanding and comprehensive inclusion of the Kototama Principle within the five life dimensions of tai kyoku allowed him to arrive at a new understanding of the Five Element diagnosis and treatment. Kototama sound deepened his understanding of the San Yin/San Yo jingei diagnosis. It allowed him to comprehend the seventeen pulses, 'the seventeen hidden gods,' that he passed to us to heal twenty-first-century planet Earth.

By the spring of 1985, the Kototama Institute had 107 graduates of its primary program and fifteen enrollees in its graduate Doctoral Program. Sensei closed the Institute's primary program and focused on his senior students. He needed to know how serious they were; they needed to know how serious he was.

He frequently told his senior students they had to "suffer" to grasp what he was teaching. Some quit the studies because they refused to adopt "suffering as part of their studies." They were too attached to their current predicament to change.

"...to suffer an experience... to be willing to be exposed to an experience that may be disturbing...to be made to think about something...to be changed in some way—at least to be forced to reconsider my perceptions, because life is very short. Why wastes your time?"
(Edward Abbey)

Some thought further studies with Osensei were a waste of time; I thought not studying with Osensei was a waste of time.

In 1984, through the efforts of many grateful and influential patients, the City of Santa Fe named him a "Living Treasure" for his cultural and spiritual contributions to the community.

In 1985, the New Mexico State Senate presented him with an Award for
Exceptional Achievement "for inspiring the passage of the New Mexico Acupuncture Practice Act."Masahilo M. Nakazono Osensei lived and breathed PASSION. He was always starving; he cried, his laugh was full, and his eyes danced and sparkled like

fireflies enjoying the delight of their existence; lessons in spoken words and lessons in silence.

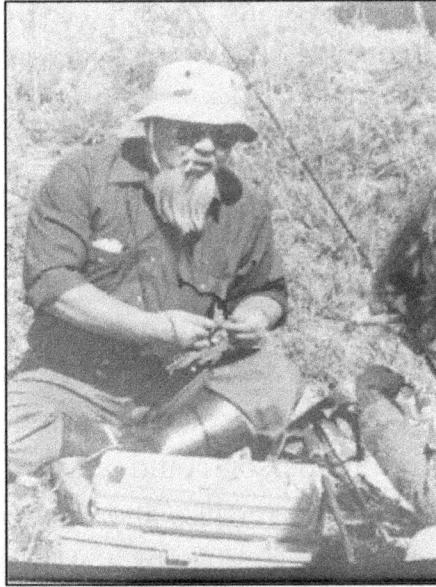

Trout   Fishing,   Heron   Lake,   NM,   circa   1983

SAKAI SENSEI

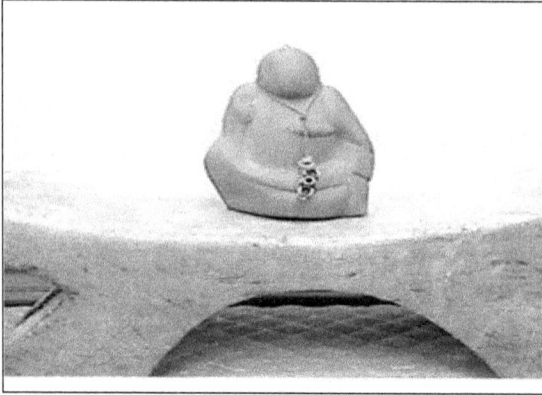

Once, a young man presented himself before Sakai, a Shugendo[4] priest, and asked for acceptance as his student. Sakai Sensei responded that this young person could not settle down to serious studies if his ancestors were restless and unattended. The would-be student expressed confusion over the master's words and pledged to be earnest. Nonetheless, Sakai Sensei dismissed him and advised him to return to his family's village and take care of his responsibilities. The young man followed these instructions, and when he arrived at the family cemetery, he found his mother's and father's tombstones knocked over. In addition, the entire family gravesite was overgrown and in general disarray.

The young man began cleaning, pruning, and planting flowers and correcting the ill-situated markers at his parent's graves. In so doing, he began to reflect on his connection to his family, past, and history.

11

[4.]The path (do) to power (gen) through ascetic practice (shu), the way of developing spiritual power, the path of cultivating psychic, spiritual, and healing powers. Shugendo is a Kami-Buddha fusion that blends mountain worship, shamanism, Shintoism, Taoism, and Buddhism. Shugenja is one who accumulates power by following the path of Shugendo.

Finally, it dawned on him that his desire to study the way of Buddha could not have happened except for all those who had gone before him. Indeed, the desire for perfection existed before he did; he was just the current manifestation of that desire. With grateful acknowledgment to his ancestors, he returned to the village where Sakai Sensei was staying to try again to gain access to his teachings; before he could make his request, Sensei accepted him into his studies.

Nakazono Osensei told this story as history, metaphor, analogy, and allegory. Sakai is asking, "Do you know what is in your head and where it originated? Do you get that you are responsible for your whole being, even your DNA?"

Master Sakai guided his students in reverence of Life Energy and its continuity through the veneration of Jizo Bosatsu, the Buddha who embodies DNA, the very fabric of our being, all that comes before us, for we are but that in the present. Jizo Bosatsu, the Buddha of uninterrupted continuation, smiles from where innocent souls and tattered spirits dwell as one, where we are never born separate. Continually acknowledging our ancestral past allows us to live in the present humbly. Our ancestors are still alive in us; therefore, we must act in the self-interest of our continually unfolding family. Modern genetic science shows how accurate Sakai Sensei was.

Masahilo M. Nakazono placed himself under the guidance of Master Sakai, renowned for his abdominal handwork in addressing physical, mental, and spiritual issues.

Master Sakai, a Buddhist priest, a wandering monk, a "mountain practicant," a yamabushi ascetic warrior who lived half the year in mountain forests, foraging his food and sleeping in caves. He was shugenja and spent half of each year living in a small village tending to the community's health needs, providing his touch as medicine while tutoring a few students in his spiritual and physical treatment practices. He diagnosed by being one with his patient; he treated through hand Qi to the abdomen.

He was a shaman who talked with animals and was reputed to be a "shape changer" who could assume the form of a white fox when necessary. However, it is not essential to these studies whether he was a "shape changer." Instead, it is more important that he was a healer who spent half of the year in a village, providing services to all in need and teaching a small group of students his way of healing through touch. Viewed as a bodhisattva, he taught that the path in the eternal present is the sum of all past actions.

Through the grace of Sakai Sensei, I provide the handwork I do. He referred to his way of healing hands as teate ('hands healing spirit'/'spiritual healing through the hands'); Masahilo M. Nakazono was Master Sakai's student. He taught him the way of spiritual hand treatment and continued guiding him until his passing in 1972. Nakazono Osensei said the proper term, based on its source, is Sakai Hon Rei Teate (Sakai's unique sacred way of healing through the hands). This "treatment by the spirit" led Sakai Sensei to unique diagnostic powers and treatment methods that he passed on to Nakazono, and now you are encountering.

Master Sakai understood the infinite spirit in finite form, Jizo Bosatsu, Earth Womb Buddha. Through Jizo Bosatsu - protector of children, expectant mothers, children who have passed before their parents, pilgrims, and travelers - that we pay homage to our roots, share our humanness, acknowledge our unity with each other, our families, our species, our planet, and the universe. Through Sakai Sensei, we gather to recognize our unity, ancestrally and socially. Through Sakai Sensei and because of Nakazono Osensei, we can experience "hands healing the spirit."

CHAPTER THREE
ENTER THE BARBARIAN

*"Do not follow in the footsteps
Of the ancient ones,
Do what they did."*

Matsuo Basho (1644-1694)

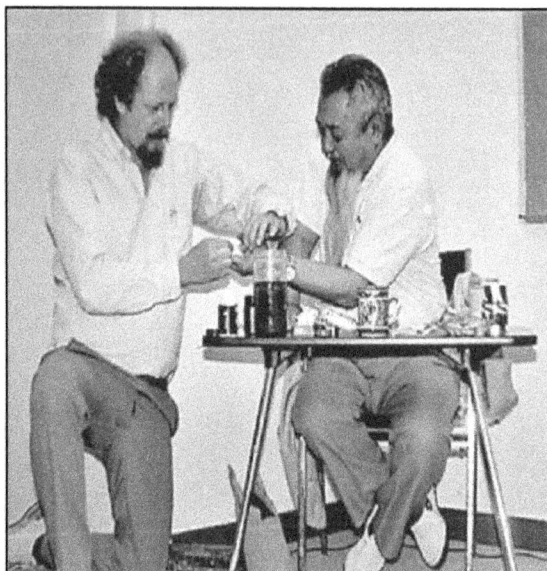

Osensei with the author, 1987

The medicine I practice is a generational transference of an evolutionary paradigm wherein the participants have no or little choice over whom partakes in the establishment of the system. As a result, an organic holism is manifesting.

My studies of the Kototama Principle began in 1973 when I read a lecture by Nakazono Osensei concerning the spiritual power of vowel-based sounds. I had been struggling for several years concerning *"why, how"* questions present with the practice of chanting, singing sacred songs, and reciting a mantra. I read his printed lectures and his books Messiah's Return and Kototama. I pondered long, challenging, and deep. The Kototama Principle might answer my question, *"How do prayer, chanting, and mantra alter consciousness?"* None of my teachers could answer this question, even those who taught me prayer, chanting, and mantra. Nothing else, no one else had answered this. I knew I had to meet him. An injury allowed that to happen.

My formal studies of traditional Japanese medicine with Masahilo Nakazono Osensei began in 1977 when he publicly taught Kototama Life Medicine. After experiencing his medicine on my immediate family members, including myself, when he saved my severely infected finger from amputation, I asked if he would take me as a student; he consented.

The Kototama Principle, the philosophical and spiritual study of the creative powers of human consciousness inherent in spoken languages, led Nakazono Osensei to recognize a new paradigm within the yin/yang, meridian, and Five Element theories. Through his quest to grasp and express the totality of human consciousness and our responsibility for human consciousness, there evolved principles and practices. These practices studied through the Kototama Principle result in a radical realignment of ancient concepts concerning diagnosis and treatment. He taught pulse diagnosis and meridian therapy on that foundation. He trained others to treat the pulses with the energetic capacity of the hands brought to maturity through daily spiritual practice. Understanding is not in needle treatment or technique alone but in guiding the pulses back to balance.

Osensei's studies and practice of Kototama brought a method of meditation to center one's spiritual journey to maintain the mental discipline necessary for the adequate delivery of acupuncture, moxibustion, and tactile therapy. Kototama medicine is not an occupation; it is a way of life. It has to do with balancing all the aspects that constitute being a living human being.

When I had completed my primary studies in 1980, Osensei invited me to join his sons on the teaching staff of the Kototama Institute. I continued my studies for the next eight years, studying and serving him continually, and remained with the Institute until it fulfilled its mission and discontinued activities in 1986.

Through Osensei, I lived a life akin to what in the Middle Ages they termed *mysterium*: education through a guild or group of dedicated people who study and practice art or skill, "secrets" known only to them, learned through years of apprenticeship, and passed on generation to generation. During the eleven years of studying with Osensei, I assisted in his revision of Inochi, The Book of Life, and the self-publishing of Guide to Inochi (Life) Medicine, a patient healthcare book developed, designed, and edited by incorporating his previous writings and lectures with my photography and synopsis of his life. Everything was handwritten many times over.

I lived for a while in my Sensei's home; I lived for a while in his clinic. I went shopping with him. I watched TV with him, primarily sports and an occasional Western. (Truly memorable: the two Saturdays spent watching twelve hours of Shogun with his extended (three generations) Nakazono family and his senior students, such laughter and learning!) I treated patients with him. I met many people with him. I went on long car rides with him. I played pool with him. I soaked in hot springs with him. I went fishing with him, where he guided me in needle technique while showing me how to catch trout. We talked. I studied. Osensei shepherded all my studies throughout those years. He guides me to this day.

My professional meridian therapy practice began in June 1980 in Santa Fe, two days after I graduated from the basic Kototama Institute program: a unique practice of classic pulse diagnosis, tactile Qi development, Japanese hari (acupuncture), okyu (moxibustion), teate (bodywork), shonishin (non-needle pediatric therapy), shokuji (diet), and self-examination—all grounded in the Kototama Principle as an integrated system of healthcare.

Comprehending the jingei diagnosis verified to Osensei the accuracy of the Kototama protocol. Understanding the jingei diagnosis is how I came to realize the dominant arrangement of the ryoku-bu-jio (wrist pulse diagnosis) is of another era, and there is another way to understand the wrist pulses. I studied the presentation of pulses relative to the jingei diagnosis and began to note pulse patterns that caused me to rethink the identity of the individual pulses. The pattern I discovered in the wrist pulses was consistent with the Sosei relationship in the Futonorito order (A I E Y O U) and the San Yin/San Yo relationship, definable through the jingei pulse. Associating the ryoku-bu-jio pulses, the San Yin/San Yo meridian relationship, and the Futonorito order of sound rhythms with a unified diagnostic understanding created a paradigm shift in pulse diagnosis, a new ryoko-bu-jio pulse pattern. In recognition of my research and findings, Osensei conferred the degree of Doctor of Kototama Life Medicine on me in 1987. From that point, I designated my approach to diagnosis and treatment as Inochi Medicine. It is the term I first used in 1986 and the pulse diagnosis method I have taught all my students since 1988. The bodywork techniques unified in this paradigm evolved and developed over the centuries and came together through the lifelong studies and practices of Osensei. Inochi (Life) Medicine became apparent through the study and practice of Kototama Life Medicine.

Inochi Medicine is an evolutionary perspective of traditional oriental medicine, establishing another pattern in the Ryokobu-jiao pulse placement, focusing on Three Yin/Three Yang diagnostics and Nakazono therapeutics. It draws on the classic Five Element meridian therapy, traditional Asian medicine, naturopathic medicine, and Kototama Life Medicine and focuses on diagnosing seventeen pulses. Treatment includes Sakai Hon Rei Teate and Kototama teate as taught by Nakazono Osensei. The application of dietary principles reflects the classic ideas of oriental medicine considering modern research. Sotai, somatic therapy, and the manual therapy techniques developed in schools of judo, kappo, and traditional and contemporary methods of critical care and folk remedies of the East and West, are all part of Inochi Medicine.

Kototama Life Medicine, Natural Life Therapy, and Inochi Medicine stand on a viewpoint that recognizes the natural rhythm of human life, and the universal rhythm of life itself are the same. Therefore, all disorders and diseases result from the disharmony of this life rhythm.

I have spent a lifetime reading the pulses, not the classics; I am neither a historian nor a researcher. I do not know any Asian languages; I am not a linguist. When asked if we should be studying Japanese, Osensei responded, "Is your life work to study languages or pulses?"

My Sensei pointed toward the classics and taught me to read living pulses. He taught me the Japanese system and instructed me to provide it to America. He encouraged me to learn the source of language, of all spoken words. Because all my studies came from traditional Japanese natural medicine, the names and terms I use come from that exposure. My studies and apprenticeship in natural medicine took place in my country and my language.

My spiritual studies emanate from holy lands and sacred spaces; my guides have been loving and demanding. My teachers have been people with the desire and capacity to share. Some are thousands of years old; I do not know the names of most. They are my professional ancestors to whom I am eternally grateful. I am thankful to those who guided Masahilo M. Nakazono Osensei, as he has guided me:

- Dr. Juzo Motoyama - acupuncture and kampo sensei
- Morihei Ueshiba Osensei - founder of aikido; messenger of Kototama sound
- Nyoichi Sakurazawa (George Ohsawa), founder of macrobiotics
- ▪ Sakai Sensei - teate master, a messenger of Jizo Bosatsu; teacher of the sacred way of hand- hara treatment.
- Koji Ogasawara Sensei - communicated the Kototama Principle; guided Nakazono Osensei in his discoveries of the relationship of Five Element meridian therapy to the Universal Energy Patterns in vocal sound.

I am most mindful and extraordinarily grateful to Masahilo M. Nakazono Osensei; he has been my life guide, healing teacher, and spiritual father. His teachings of consciousness expansion have guided me through Kototama sound, its relationship within the five dimensions of Tai Kyoku[5], the discernable qualities of Life Energy realized through the seventeen pulses, and San Yin/San Yo - the three aspects of Life Energy.

I share what I have learned, what's been revealed, what I know, what's fun to write about, and what I feel is essential. I share it as a travel log, diary, biography, textbook, workbook, recipe book, and road map. Its design serves the studies of those seeking to grasp the work of Masahilo M. Nakazono Osensei, his contributions to understanding the Five Element source, his guidance in Kototama Principle, and his guidance in my understanding of pulse diagnosis.

This information is for family, friends, physicians, priests, and students. It was initiated by experiences with Masahilo M. Nakazono and forty years of study and practice of Kototama Life Medicine. I write this to ensure that more people have access to practitioners who are students of pulse diagnosis and to assure our ancestors that pulse diagnosis will continue through ongoing studies, practice, refinement, and evolution of consciousness. I am writing this to reach the next generation of practitioners.

I am sharing what I consider the Holy Grail, the capacity to be in union with the energy of Life, the energy of the Universe, through the pulses. I hope this will inspire discussion and further study of all healing aspects and the healing process.

---

5 Chinese tai chi. The void, supreme ultimate, center between heaven and earth.

Osensei told the students of the Kototama Institute that they could earn a doctorate by studying with him for ten years and demonstrating active participation in the conversation. When I presented my thesis concerning a reinterpretation of ryoku-bujio, my clinical findings, and our joint clinical provings, he designed his diploma He commissioned Kazuo Chiba Sensei, a Japanese Aikido master, calligrapher, and longtime personal and professional associate of Osensei's, to provide the calligraphy for the diploma. He made four degrees in Japanese and English: the first one to his first-born son; the second to his younger son; the third to his longtime aikido/acupuncture student in France, and the fourth degree he presented to me at a gathering of his senior students from North America and Europe. First, he acknowledged my research and explained our conclusions. Then, he suggested they further research this paradigm, told his audience I was useless, and presented me with his endorsement. Thank you, Sensei.

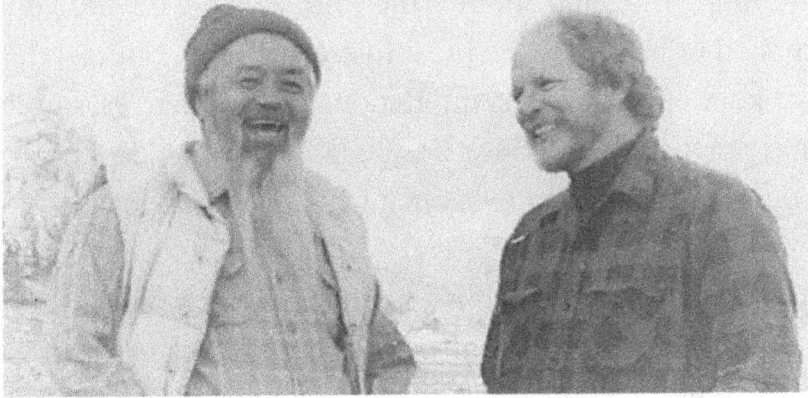

Masahilo M. Nakazono   Thomas E. Duckworth,
Colorado Fishing Trip, 1983

CHAPTER FOUR
ETHOS

Humans have suffered from disease and trauma since the beginning of existence and simultaneously have sought remedies and techniques to reduce suffering. As experience and knowledge accumulated, medicine developed from initial instinctive treatment.

Laying on of hands started about the time hands appeared on bodies. When we were young and injured, we covered the wound with our hand and pressed. We did not know that pressure allows the blood to clot, which stops the bleeding. We did know that it relieves pain and usually prevents post trauma achiness. We did not know that pressure would relieve blunt trauma injuries and even the pain of broken bones, that it reduces inflammation, stimulates lymphatic activity, slows the heart rate, slows the breathing rate, and soothes the soul. When we were young, we rubbed or held the "ouchie." In our memory, our (O) dimension, we held on to these accumulations of experiences, observations, and practical logic. Such has been the case since the very beginning of human existence when hands appeared.

There are primal, instinctive actions to which we have always had access. Other creatures also instinctively act in their selfinterest concerning healthcare. Bears rub against trees; cats lick themselves; rabbits scratch themselves; bovines nibble on a bush to address skin cancer; dogs eat grass for digestive issues. At first, we can assume that treatments were intuitive and experiential. As our prehistoric ancestors experienced individual and collective actions of care and preservation, the brain evolved, memory accumulated, and the healing arts developed. Variances worldwide in geography, climate, culture, language, and experience have resulted in the development of various systems of medicine.

Undoubtedly, massage is the oldest form of organized "laying on of hands," and every culture has developed or copied styles, techniques, and protocols of healing touch. We have always grasped the benefits of touch. We have created whole professions and social structures to allow and encourage the "laying on of hands." Bodyworkers, magicians, physicians, priests, shamans, midwives, nurses, and acupuncturists have employed touch as a healing method for many thousands of years. Burmese practitioners were adjusting hips and backs and addressing other structural alignments a thousand years before bio-mechanical was a word. Chiropractic began by observing Chinese laborers building the Transcontinental Railroad, performing ancient massage and tactile therapy on each other. If you need your neck adjusted in the Philippines, you go to the barber.

Historically, the second oldest form of healthcare—trauma care—developed and evolved through warfare. From the earliest medical writings and traditions of the ancient cultures, there are instructions addressing avulsions, abrasions, lacerations, punctures, fractures, dislocations, soft tissue injuries, burns, drowning, shock, anger, fear, hysteria, depression, poisoning, infections, sore muscles, fatigue and more. We have always been able to hurt each other. However, we are still searching for ways to assist each other. The Napoleonic Wars included the invention of the ambulance.

In Japan, an entire system of osteopathic care and trauma medicine – kappo - developed through the study and practice of judo. Certified practitioners were referred to as "bone setters", and by the late nineteenth century, the profession was an honored therapeutic practice provided by judo practitioners holding the rank of third dan. Masahilo M. Nakazono Osensei was certified in Kappo prior to World War II.

Part of our evolutionary data gathering includes the usage of plants, animals, and mineral substances for external and internal applications. We collectively have discovered and developed remedies in the form of teas, gargles, and flushes that we chew, swallow, inhale, rub, soak, or apply as a poultice or compress, which grow in our backyard, barnyard, forests, and far away. Cultures share, and healing arts evolved around the principle of hands-on medicine.

Some of our collective knowledge represents our capacity to understand the appropriateness of rubbing a cold arm; some of our collective understanding represents our capacity to understand yin/yang. Some of our collective experience comes from grandma; some comes from people with a life-long dedication to discovering and transmitting healing ways. The Japanese, Persians, Indians, Chinese, Greeks, and others have been quite extensive in their research, writings, and ability to pass on profound information to future generations. Before written languages, the ancestors spoke their knowledge and wisdom.

Oral and visual transmissions of the healing ways are still prime ingredients in the learning environment. Much of the information that needs dissemination involves spoken words and hands-on demonstrations. If books like this one could teach, we would all be great masters—books record stuff. People who empower their path through at least ten years of study, practice, awe, humility, humor, dedication, and complete acceptance of studenthood may acquire the capacity to teach. To teach, one must spend years learning empirical knowledge. Talking about someone else's knowledge is not teaching, nor is it knowledge.

Ming medicine came to Japan from China in the early sixth century. Years later, medical codes established educational standards and the ranks of teacher and practitioner. The code required seven years of schooling and training for internal medicine and seven years of study of diagnosis and treatment by needling and moxibustion. Both pediatrics and surgery required five years of training; ear/eye/throat specialists trained for four years. Successful completion of training earned a Master of Medicine degree in the respective specialty. However, it took considerable postgraduate clinical experience to qualify for the title of Doctor of Medicine and earn the right to teach. Fourteen hundred years later, it is still understood the journey from practitioner to teacher is at least a decade long.

Different cultures, different schools of thought, different practitioners focus on various unique facets and approaches to healing. In all cultures and traditions, a serious practitioner will spend decades in clinical studies and practice to comprehend one aspect of that healing art. The practitioner dedicated to the mastery of hari, the diagnostic and treatment principles of acupuncture, cannot also be studying to master the diagnostic and treatment principles of Kampo[13] if actual mastery is the goal in either discipline.

One might be a good acupuncturist and a good herbalist but never achieve the expert skills that come through focused attention to a "Way," the Tao of one medicine. Osensei taught us teate. He did not follow a book or a method. He trained to perform general handwork by light rubbing with the fingers straight, palm, and fingers flat; he did not name this technique "keisatsu." Appaku: applying hand or thumb pressure on the body's surface, but not deep, addressing tendons, ligaments, and the connections of bones, joints, and muscles is a technique he taught without naming. Shinsen: vibrating nerves and muscles with the palm or finger; Annetsu: squeezing and kneading with fingers or thumb with a circular, vertical pressure for affecting bones, joints, and connective tissue; Junetsu, soft kneading with a firm grip for massaging muscle; Koda, tapping with the side of the fist, "soft fist: or knuckles for affecting the nervous system.

---

13) Japanese traditional herbal medicine, refined in the seventeenth century by Yoshimasu,Todo. He developed a refined technique of abdominal palpation, fukushin, to provide additional information in determining the appropriate herbal formula.

All were taught as one continuous expression of teate, touching diagnosis, and therapy of Qi.

After I was in practice for a few years, I saw some books on Shiatsu and Anma and discovered that the healing touch had been defined, systematized, copyrighted, and certified. I was taught Teate.

"The activity of the universe continually manifests out through the human seed. There are five types of energy. These energies form and hold the body together. They flow as currents, meridians, through the human seed, manifesting this energy before creating organs. Organs manifest this energy, as do blood and whole systems. All the currents should be in balance. Each current must have its power. Each current is different, not the same. The energy necessary to manifest the individual organs is different. Each organ's volume, size, and density vary; therefore, the current varies.
Nakazono Osensei, class notes, July 20, 1977

"This energy: moving, dynamic, spiraling in all directions - connect, and form manifests. These places are where form manifests. The human body is acting from universal energy. So, the way of the medicine is to ask the question, which meridians have lost their balance? Which meridian is affecting the other meridians? Then, balance that meridian.
Nakazono Osensei, class notes, July 20, 1977

"The total 'volume' of energy, the full capacity of this energy, expresses as five 'negative' and five 'positive' meridians manifesting aposteriori organs and five 'negative' and five 'positive' meridians manifesting apriori energies. These twenty meridians synchronize with each other and produce life in the form."
Nakazono Osensei, class notes, July 20, 1977

Apriori (cannot see),
Aposteriori (can see),
We can only see one side.

"The opposite of everything is always manifesting.
An atom has opposite energy. We cannot see it.
Apriori determines aposteriori."

Nakazono Osensei, class notes

Meridians
10 Aposteriori
   (in form)

20
Energy has a meridian, a pulse,
   and an associated organ and is
   paired.

Liver (Lv) Gallbladder (GB)
Heart (Ht)   Small Int. (SI)
Lung (Lu) ......Large Int. (LI)
Kidney (Kd) ...Bladder (Bl)
Spleen (Sp)   Stomach (St)

10 Apriori
(before form)

2 - Energy has a meridian and a pulse but does not manifest as an organ.

    Shimpo ((HC)
    Sansho (TH)

2 – Energy has a meridian but does not have a pulse or manifest as an organ.

    Toku (GV)   Nin (CV)

6 - Energy shares meridians, has no pulse, does not manifest as an organ

    Sho, Tai, Yin Yi, Yo Yi,
    Yin Kyo, Yo Kyo

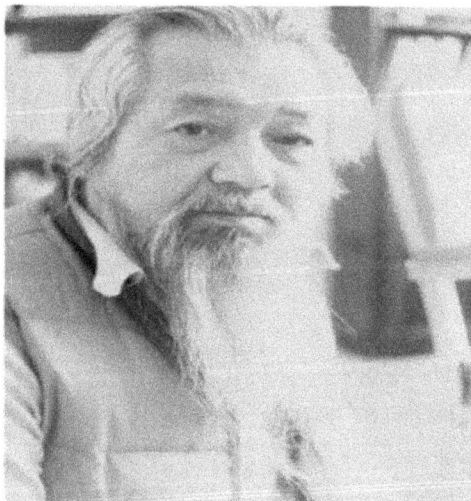

CHAPTER FIVE

KOTOTAMA PRINCIPLE

The practice of Kototama Life Medicine is a return to the original principle; universal life manifesting itself.

There are various schools of traditional oriental medicine. There are differing points of view on the actions and functions of meridians, differing values of the four aspects of diagnosis, differing interpretations of pulse diagnosis, differing significance to the body-mind-spirit phenomenon and changing "sense and sensibilities" concerning the "classics."

The study and understanding of acupuncture evolve within the cultural, linguistic, social, and ecological environment in which it is practiced. Not only are there distinct demarcations of "Chinese" acupuncture and "Japanese" acupuncture, but it is also becoming evident there is evolving "American" acupuncture. Within this newly changing paradigm, the influences of the classics will differ as they are restudied and applied anew. Even the sense of what the classics are may be redefined.

Kototama medicine brings the theory of the Five Elements closer to the law of the Five Elements. Development involved studying the classics, the I Ching and the Kojiki, the form of language and information from lost texts, such as the Takenouchi Documents and the Dead Sea Scrolls, as well as the discoveries of modern science. Kototama Life Medicine seeks the present moment, Naka-ima, 'now- here.'

Kototama Natural Life Therapy-Inochi Medicine is a system that recognizes the healing capacity inherent within the energetic form and function of the body. Within this system, the power of human life is distinguished and influenced via a dynamic web, meridians, by a unified creative, vital force termed Qi. Thus, the study of energetic patterns and their relationships and usage affect the overall harmony of Life Energy. This harmony synchronizes human life's will-to-be, decision-to-be, spirit-of-being, form-ofbeing, and continuity-of-being. In the language of our studies, these aspects of Life Energy are the foundational sound pulses: I, E, A, U, O. In explaining the influence of meridians in reestablishing harmony and synchronization, the meridian of blood circulation, the meridian of air/gas circulation, the meridian of purification, the meridian of nutrition, and the meridian of water circulation are cited. These dimensions of human beingness have come to be awkwardly termed fire/heart, metal/lung, wood/liver, earth/spleen, and water/kidney.

The Kototama Principle expressed in OA (*mind/spirit),* the intellectual expression of the spiritual dimension, established a mission through the writings and public teachings of Professor Koji Ogasawara of Tokyo, Japan, who founded Dai San Bummei Kai (The Third Civilization Association). He taught from the 1940s until he died in 1979. Through studying the basic sounds of human language, he sought to clarify the concept of the grand unifying principle of human consciousness within spoken words to express the unity of the universe. He taught, *"The voice is the selfexpression of life."* Reality exists through the human expression of it. This expression creates a consciousness within the framework of three arrangements of actuality, "three civilizations" identified by Ogasawara Sensei as the three archetypes of personal and social selfcreation.

Three civilizations are the three societies, mentalities, formed by the expression of Sugaso, Kanagi, or Futonorito orders of language.

The <u>First Civilization</u>, <u>Sugaso</u> order, manifests through the sound pattern: A O U E I. It expresses the life spirit (A) continually (O) shining on lifeform (U), empowering (E) the search for the soul of existence (I). The spirit realm (A) leads by the Judgement of Spirit, AE dimension. Archetype: Elder, Guide, Missionary, Physician, Poet, Priest. One who seeks unification.

The <u>Second Civilization</u>, <u>Kanagi</u> order, manifests the sound rhythm: A I U E O. Spirit (A) recognizes soul (I) within form (U), judging (E) that (U) as central and holds that mentally, in memory (O). It guides through the physical-mental (UO) dimension. It voices the light of life (A) shining on the life-will (I) of the physical dimension (U), empowers (E), and continues (O); this is the scientific-materialistic realm OU. Archetype:

Academic, Banker, Lawyer, Politician, Educationalist, Technician, Theologian, Soldier. One who creates boundaries, borders, distinctions, hierarchies, restrictions, and separation.

<u>The Third Civilization</u>, <u>Futonorito</u> order, manifests A I E O U. Spirit (A) recognizing soul (I) accepts power (E) continually (O) ennobling form (U). This consciousness administers from IE, lifewill/life-judgment. The light of life (A) illuminates' life-will (I)

55

and expresses life power (E) and life memory (O) in the life form (U). It is the unification of spirit and material, soul, and body. Archetype: Younger Citizen/Senior Citizen. One who unites.

One aspect of this consciousness-shifting journey is viewed as an evolutionary process through time. We had an ancient era when we communicated with each other (First Civilization), followed by our current period where communication is self-centered (Second Civilization). Now, our collective consciousness seeks to create a realization of unity, developing the best aspects of the First and Second civilizations through the (IE) dimension of the Third Civilization. A new consciousness forms because "you can't step in the same river twice."

Another aspect is identifiable within our being. These three orders of consciousness (civilizations) are each of us. We exhibit aspects of being full of light and spirit in the physical world while seeking our soul (AUI), Sugaso order, and we can live, think, and behave in ego (UEO), Kanagi order. However, human consciousness, life-will, and life-action (IE) seek to harmonize these aspects of human capacity and do so within the Futonorito order.

This consciousness-shifting journey is horizontal in that it is within a long history; it is vertical in that the First, Second, and Third civilizations exist within, perpetually, Nakaima. We choose what reality in which we are living. We establish it, reinforce it, and define it with our words. Words express the reality we wish to live in or mistakenly believe the only option we have.

To Ogasawara Sensei, the spiritual sense of "we are all one" and the religious sense that "we are made in the image and likeness of God" are truths that need much more in-depth understanding if we are to reunite the world population.

Koji Ogasawara Sensei shared his grasp of the Kototama (Word Soul) Principle through writing, publishing, and leading the Third Civilization Association and its monthly study group regarding the journey into the Third Civilization. In *The Passage To The Third Civilization*, he acknowledged over twenty individual scholars, researchers, writers, teachers, and students who had contributed to his studies and understanding of the unity of body and soul. For years, Masahilo Nakazono was a very attentive student. They never met. They wrote letters.

The Kototama (Word Soul) Principle is expressed in the AU dimension (*spirit form*) through Ueshiba Osensei, who created Aikido within his studies of the Kototama Principle of sound energy and sought to guide us back to our center, back to SU.

The Kototama Principle conveyed in AIE dimension (*spirit/life/action*) acquired a representation through the research, writings, and public teachings of Dr. Masahilo M. Nakazono Osensei, who uncovered the Kototama Futonorito order of meridian therapy. He founded the Kototama Institute to teach Kototama Life Medicine as an expression of the Kototama Principle.

This system expresses the Kototama Principle. Kototama sound, integrated with Sakai hand Qi through SU, allows Qi's energetic assimilation and dissemination through the hands. Sakai Hon Rei Teate, modifying energetic stagnation and inflammation of mind, body, and spirit through hand Qi expression to the abdomen, coupled with Nakazono teate that includes anma, ampuku, shiatsu, Nakazono kappo, and sotai. Diagnosis and treatment are expressions of the capacity of the hands.

Nakazono Osensei taught the Kototama sound principle, pulse diagnosis, hand Qi development, and meridian therapy. The

Kototama Principle is the map; hand Qi enhancement, pulses, meridians, and tsubo are the avenues we travel. The tools are varied. The student of Kototama medicine begins the study of acupuncture after demonstrating the ability to alter the energy manifesting through the pulses, first with teate ("hands healing spirit"), then with kyu (moxibustion). After a focused period of training the hands to access Qi from tanden, combined with intensive studies of pulses in guiding teate and kyu Qi therapy, hari (acupuncture) studies begin. Always the student is guided toward Qi. We are all studying.

"When you step back far enough into yourself, you will come to the void, having no beginning and no end. It is the center of the universe and the self-manifests from there to here-now. Theoretical science recognizes the void as the 'center' of the physical world, yet it is the source of our being."

(class notes)

Acupuncture is a verb. Acupuncture is not just needling; it is the art and science of influencing the body's life energy to bring about specific changes in a person's health.

This includes the entire realm of the healing arts and clinical applications that recognize the world and the human body as statements of the universe. The laws that govern the expression of the universe are the same that govern human life. They are singular yet universal. This wholeness in each part extends to the realm of diagnosis and treatment. Sticking a needle in a person is not acupuncture; diagnosing and treating according to the laws of Qi is acupuncture. It includes needle, moxibustion, herbal and dietary therapy, tactile therapy, psychotherapy, spiritual therapy, and compassion. Acupuncture is the whole experience of care.

Life Energy termed "the electromagnetic energy of the body," is more than that. It is the elemental energy of the universe recognized by physicists as the constituent energy of all formation. It is the fundamental interface of nature: gravitational force, electromagnetic force, weak force, strong force, and the Grand Unified Theory. It is called Life Energy (vital force in English), ki or tai kyoku in Japanese, chi or Qi in Chinese, ansuz in Old Norse, prana in Sanskrit.

Life energy, Qi, consists of five fundamental factors necessary for life: desire-to-be (A), will-to-be (I), power-to- be (E), the continuation of being (O), and form of being (U). This vital force/Life Energy encompasses all actions of being: emotional power (A), spiritual power (I), judgment power (E), mental power (O), physical power (U); all physical senses of being: sight (A), touch (I), smell (E), listening (O), taste (U); and all spiritual senses of being: emotion (A), inspiration (I), aspiration (E) intuition (O), universal spirit (U). Disorder in any aspect of our being is a sign of blockage or fatigue of Qi. The remedy is to liberate obstructed Qi and enhance depleted Qi

These blockages result in energy deficiencies: yang jitsu, excessive energy expanding without judgment, and yin jitsu, exhausted energy trapped and unable to move. Yin kyo, not drawing power nor holding power, results in stagnation of blood, fluids, air, nutrition, and yang kyo, unable to freely transport, results in depletion of protective Qi, nutritive Qi, and vital Qi.

Meridian therapy, like physics, recognizes that form exists because of energy. Therefore, if a form is out of balance, the problem arises from energy out of balance. Revitalize the energy, and the form will follow. Do not get sidetracked by dysfunction of form and function; do not chase after symptoms. In its totality, the body responds to the expression of its energy.

The body becomes stiff when there is stagnation of blood and other fluids. Stiffness exerts abnormal pressure on nerves, circulatory, lymph, digestive, and skeletal systems. Therapy not only releases blockages but allows the individual to become aware of the blocked or tense areas of one's body. Influence the body without trauma to reinstate Qi's flow, allowing the body to reestablish homeostasis.

Satisfactory results from treatment happen when the four aspects of diagnosis, tsubo location and selection, and the treatment of enhance (ho) and liberate (sha) combine properly. The most important is palpating the tsubo and treating while dwelling in tanden. This may require years of practice.

The studies begin with hand Qi exercise, the union of mind-body-spirit through focused attention to breathing and Qi as exemplified in the discoveries of Ueshiba Osensei, founder of aikido, the teachings of Sakai Sensei, and the work of M.M. Nakazono Osensei. Hand Qi exercise is the center of our meditation, tactile therapy, moxibustion, and acupuncture.

Kototama Natural Life Medicine includes
Ampuku (traditional Japanese abdominal diagnosis and treatment)
- **Go Gyo, anma, and shiatsu** (Five Element tactile healing)
- **Jingei** (carotid artery) diagnosis
- **Kei raku chiryo** (meridian therapy)
- **Kototama Go Gyo** (Kototama Five Element principles)
- **Kototama Sound** meditation and therapeutics
- **Nakazono kappo** (muscular/skeletal revitalization therapy)
- **Roku gyo** dietary guidance: sour, bitter, pungent, umami/savory, salt, sweet
- **Ryoku-bu-jio-yi** (both hands, six pulses) diagnosis.
- **Sakai Hon Rei Teate** (Qi-centric abdominal handwork developed by Sakai Sensei)
- **Sota**i (muscle reprogramming therapy)

Kototama Inochi Medicine evolved as a system of healthcare in which diagnosis by the wrist and neck pulses are central to the application of the remedy. The principles of treatment, grounded in implementing the Kototama Principle, adhere to traditional methods and concepts. The therapy system incorporates handwork, manipulative therapy, diet and exercise, movement, centering techniques, acupuncture, moxibustion, and psyche-spiritual therapy. The students of Kototama medicine correct pulse conditions with their hands before they learn acupuncture techniques. They know how to guide a person's diet by reading the pulses, and they work on themselves before they work on another. Kototama Life Medicine is not a system of acupuncture. It is a lifecare system based on the individual's pure energetics as observed in the pulses; therapy may take many forms.

Kototama Inochi Medicine is an ever inclusive method of healthcare that represents the self-worth of life, the dignity of the individual, and the boundless capacity of the human to synchronize with the Will and Power creating and sustaining life itself.

This linage, the Kototama way of myaku (the pulse), involves interpreting the twelve pulses, termed ryoku-bu- jio-yi in the three wrist positions sunko, kanjo, and shaku- chu, plus Chu Myaku (the Life Pulse/middle pulse/'stomach' pulse) and jingei-myakuko, the pulse at Lower Yo Mei (St) # 9
(Jingei).

From nothing comes one, tai kyok7u; therefore, two, yin/yang, and the five elements necessary for the existence of life: life-will-to-be, life-decision-to-be, life-spirit-to-be, life-form-in-being, life-continuation-of being. In modern times, oriental medicine refers to this cosmic dance of creation as the Five Element theory. It seeks to persuade wood, fire, earth, metal, and water to improve their interactions. In Kototama Inochi Medicine, these essential five ingredients of life formation are manifestations of the primary sound rhythms created as the finite universe begins. The universe enunciates its presence and identifies itself through the human voice. This is the key. The universe manifests the human as its voice uttering, "I am." The universe, One, is partitioned by words; our intellect separates and defines with words. Phenomena come into reality through words.

It is the human being who names phenomena. We bring about separation with language. The five vowel sounds, the five elements, and the five pairs of aposteriori meridians are all manifestations of the same universal Life Energy.

The spirit of being, including its mobility, equilibrium, and preservation, is the (A) dimension, the spirit awakening, Ketsu Yin/Sho Yo. Those who name it "liver meridian" or "wood element" look at the symbolism and take analogy as reality. What is termed the "wood element" is, in fact, the human soul.

Such studies of sound rhythms and vibratory phenomena manifesting as meridians are lengthy. Nakazono Osensei recognized the five vowel sounds found worldwide in languages and the Five Elements universal in life are the same vibrational force. This recognition changes how one speaks and treats meridians, regardless of language or lineage.

Chu Myaku pulse provides the feedback of the aposteriori meridians plus the apriori meridians, Shimpo/Sansho, via pulsations within Chu Myaku. Traditionally, these six zo and six fu aspects of Life Energy are the elements: wood, fire, fire minister, earth, metal, and water. Treatment models based on the traditional

Five Element theory described different relationships among the meridians, including the creative, so-sei, motherchild relationship and the controlling, Sokoku, grandparent-grandchild relationship. This paradigm has guided many practitioners for many years with significant successes.

Within the understanding of Kototama, these six zo and six fu aspects of Life Energy are dimensions: (A)-spirit, (I)will, (E)-power, (Y)-source, (O)continuation, (U)-form and presents a treatment protocol of So Sei (mother-child) relationship. (A) dimension (liver) is the child of (U) dimension (spleen), and mother of (I) dimension (heart); (I) dimension is the child of (A), and the mother of (E) dimension (lung); (E) dimension is the child of (I) dimension and mother of (YI) dimension (fire minister/Shimpo – 'source'). (YI) dimension is the child of (E) and mother of (O) dimension (kidney), which is the child of (YI) and mother of (U) dimension (spleen); which is the child of (O) and the mother of (A). This approach to diagnosis and treatment is enhanced through jingei diagnosis.

Familial Relationships of the Six Zo/Six
Fu Myaku Kototama Inochi Paradigm

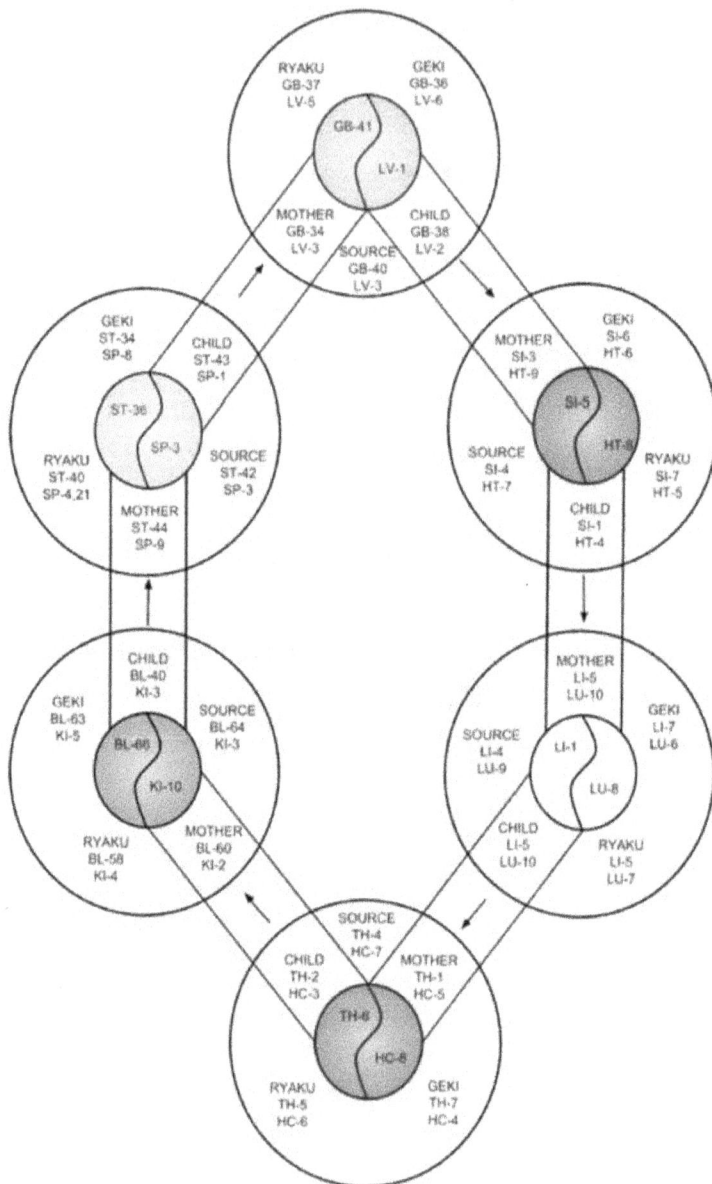

Five Element Relationship (Kanagi)

The current paradigm – wood, fire, earth, metal, water – the
Kanagi Order of Energetics

Kototama sound pattern – A, I, U, E, O

Traditional Five Element
Pattern
Kanagi Order

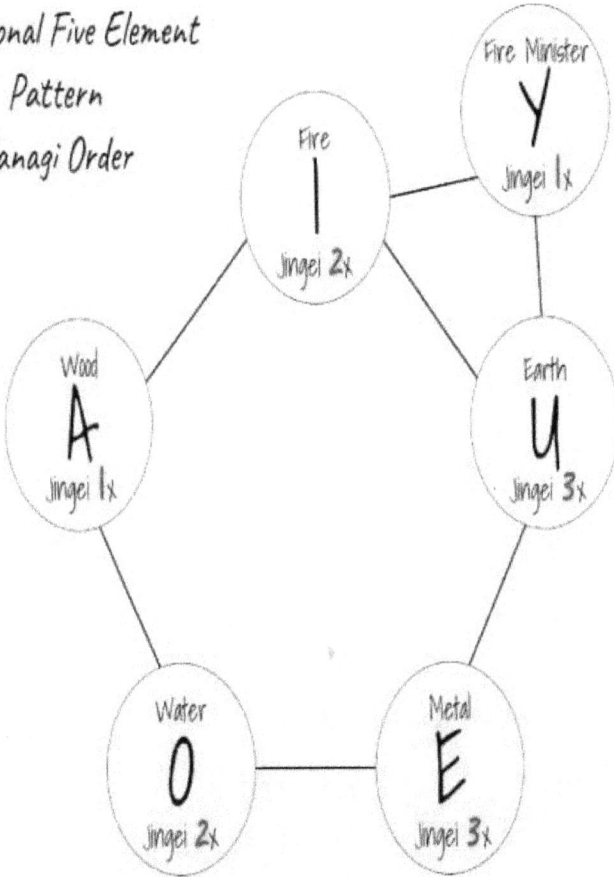

Fire Minister
Y
Jingei 1x

Fire
I
Jingei 2x

Wood
A
Jingei 1x

Earth
U
Jingei 3x

Water
O
Jingei 2x

Metal
E
Jingei 3x

Five Element Relationship (Futonorito)

Futonorito order of energetics, the new paradigm – wood, fire, metal, water, earth.

Kototama sound pattern - A, I, E, O, U

Kototama Five Element Pattern
Futnorito Order

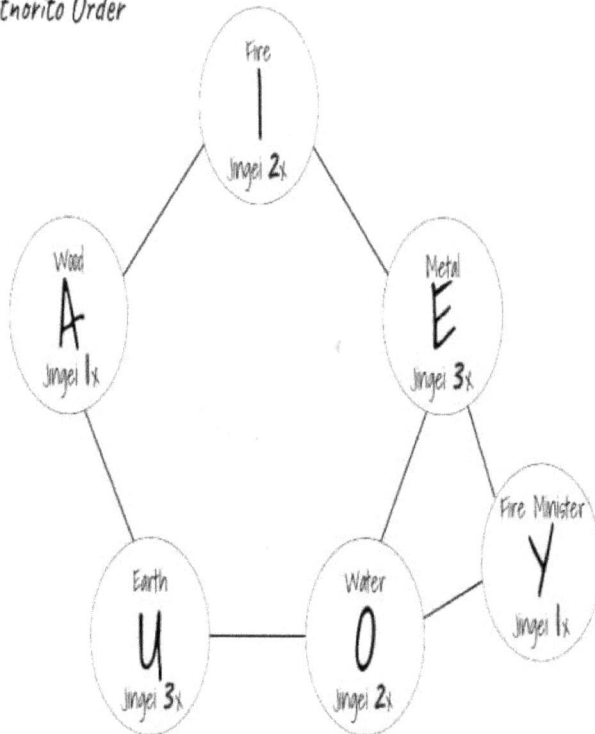

Fire
I
Jingei 2x

Wood
A
Jingei 1x

Metal
E
Jingei 3x

Fire Minister
Y
Jingei 1x

Earth
U
Jingei 3x

Water
O
Jingei 2x

Traditionally there are twenty primary meridians: twelve main meridians and eight extraordinary meridians. All meridians are extraordinary. There are ten aposteriori (formed) meridians and ten apriori (before form) meridians. As one deepens the study of Kototama, it becomes clear that this is more than semantics. The order and connectedness of body-mind-spirit within all living beings, the thinking process of the mind, and the spiritual development of all humanity can be understood through the Kototama Principle and utilized in meridian therapy.

The Kototama Principle considers the essence of being human manifests as language—creating art, science, social intercourse, philosophy, agriculture, and medicine—and the human can attune to the order and logic of the creative force. Thus, as individuals, we may understand and act by this principle of universal harmony.

The principle of Kototama focuses on the essential elements of creation manifest by the five vowel sounds of language. This principle of creation within the sound is consistent with the Five Element theory of traditional oriental medicine and serves as a cornerstone of Kototama medicine. Nakazono Osensei discovered that treating patients corresponding to Kototama Futonorito Five Element principles had results more beneficial than following the traditional Kanagi order[4] of the flow of the elemental energies.

This universal rhythm manifests in the meridians. The pulses discovered through traditional oriental medicine are the indicators of the synchronicity of this energy. Understanding what these pulses indicate is within the studies of Kototama. The proficiency in the diagnostic pulse at Lower Yo Mei (St) #9 (Jingei) enhances understanding of the subtler aspects of the wrist pulse diagnosis.

The practice of Kototama Inochi Medicine, while based on the principles of sound pulse and understanding of the seventeen

---

[4] A, I, U, E, O: wood, fire, earth, metal, water; liver, heart, spleen, lung, kidney

pulses, draws on healing techniques developed over time, including

1.   Sakai Hon Rei Teate: the soft tissue abdominal treatment form taught by the Shugendo monk, Sakai Sensei.

2.   Hari and kyu: Traditional Japanese acupuncture and moxibustion.

3.   Anma (massage), shiatsu (tactile meridian therapy), and sotai (muscular reprogramming). .

4.   Kappo: the muscular/skeletal restoration therapy that arose through the art of judo

5.   Traditional dietary and herbal healing practices, including aspects of macrobiotics, were developed by Professor George Ohsawa, and refined by Nakazono Osensei while he was Dr. Ohsawa's student.

6.   Appreciation of simplicity

CHAPTER SIX

QI DEVELOPMENT

THE HEALER

The Healer is each person's Life Energy in the form of meridians, organs, systems, spirit, mind, and persona. We assist or facilitate the Healer's ability, karma, and self-determination. Stay dedicated to one's own body. We are more centered when we can maintain a balance between the giver and the receiver. First, work on oneself before touching another. If you are weak, tired, or ill, both sessions will be unsatisfactory. If your diet is full of dense proteins, your attitude may be tense, tight, and aggressive; it may be challenging for your client to listen to their problems honestly. The treatment may be harsh. If your diet is too light or is full of sugar, oils, and processed foods, you may not be able to concentrate. Without focus, it is easy to get depressed or negative. Practice centering, meditation, concentration, and breathing at the beginning of each day. Get in touch with your hands, through your hands. Breathe. Breathe rhythmic, deep, slow breaths from your tanden.

Purposefully coordinate your breath with your patient, allowing for relaxation. You can alter your client's breathing with your own. Breath is the first action. The second action is LOVE. St. Paul: "If a person does all the right things but has not love, it is all for nothing." (Thank you, Krishna Das, for reminding me of St. Paul's reminder.) The one you must love first is yourself. You must take care of yourself as you would take care of someone you love.

Spirit healing is not an esoteric concept, nor a spiritual phenomenon available only to the initiate, nor is it of religion, nor casual bodies. Every one of us is living and manifests living energy. We are studying the energy of the form and the conscious "tapping into" that energy through deliberate actions of the structure itself.

When working with another, the active delivering participant uses the body as a channel rather than a vehicle; the receptive accepting partner has a body that is a field of energy (energy as a form) disharmonious to itself. The active member's body acts from within its source; it does nothing, but the hands move, and there is something. It is the spirit of the hand.

The way is through focus, not knowledge, and the way to focus is to change how your mind operates. Make your way to that place where you create mind changes and change your mind. On what are you centered? If you have not yet found what to center on, you are still in your old mindset; you have not changed your mind. Focused, you are not. Try softer; focus without effort. The place of focus for the hands is the Sea of Qi, three finger widths below the navel. You do NOTHING with your body; you receive intuition, insight, inspiration, and Qi through your hands. The more you receive, the more you retain; the more you hold, the more you will know because it will be your acquired knowledge. *"It's yours"* means *"it is you."* To obtain such knowledge, one must let go of all experience not coming from hand. Know nothing, seek nothing, do nothing, gain attentiveness to energy.

Osensei always stressed unceasing practice and studies: "You cannot develop intuition. But you can practice your training and master basic skills. Only through sincere long-time practice will intuition develop."\

Osensei taught us to function within tanden, seeing through our hands and perceiving energy patterns.

> *"We are not treating symptoms, not even treating the physical constitution; we are facilitating the person's own Life Energy. Only each person can heal oneself. We can assist; we must do our best. However, if we think we can cure, then we are saying that we are God, that we can create life, create a cell or an organ. Cannot. Never tell someone you can cure them; don't tell them you can help. Just say, 'I will do my best.'"*
>
> Masahilo M. Nakazono, class notes

Osensei spoke of being able to treat both sides, Ho (Enhance) and Sha (Liberate), through the power of our hands.

Enhance: Replenish deficient Qi. Other schools label it Ho.

Liberate: Disperse excessive Qi. Other schools label it Sha.

Osensei told a story about a young boy in France who had 'magical' power in his left hand. Just by his touch, he could cure, sometimes, but only with his left hand; his right hand had no influence. He could only, sometimes, fix some conditions. There was no balance. He had power but could only address one side of an imbalance; yin/yang, kyo, or jitsu, we do not know, but clearly, there was a disconnect between his "left" and "right" sides.

71

Many years ago, I worked with a First Citizen, Hopi Nation, who had acquired a healing touch after being struck by lightning but had no control of this capability. She could not influence her energetic contribution's force, flow, or dosage. But, introduced to the place and space of tanden and hand Qi exercise, she self-resolved the dynamic disconnects and could share her gift consciously.

The healing begins with the patient's trust in the practitioner and treatment method. For the person to have that kind of confidence, especially initially, they must sense your inner faith in yourself. You trust yourself through your actions, movements, and inner demeanor, and the healing begins.

We start with our hands energizing, becoming conscious, reaching down into the Sea of Qi, and sounding out from the original sound and space of separation, the first-born place of named phenomena. Health involves the many factors and functions of body/mind/spirit synergized. Ill health, disease, and dysfunction result from a lack of synergy of body/mind/spirit. To work on "other," one must always be working on self.

MISOGI (purification)
(first shared by Masahilo M. Nakazono in
*Kan'nagara (*Great Mind*), 1972*)

Qi development includes misogi[16], the purification of mind and body.

<u>External</u> <u>purification</u> consists of rubbing the body with water to wash away grime. _____

16 Ueshiba Osensei, the founder of aikido, explained misogi this way: "**MI** represents both the body and the mind, the outer and inner aspects of a human being; **SO** is ample development (memory) of **SU**, the Divine Spark; and **GI** (Qi) stands for whiteness that is clear and untainted. In **misogi,** one returns to the very beginning, where there is no differentiation between oneself and the universe."

Internal purification detoxifies the inner organs through deep breathing (breath exercise).

Spiritual purification embraces cleansing the heart through silence/sounds and mantras to rid oneself of maliciousness.

Physical preparation:

a) Sit in half or full lotus position or zazen, kneeling on the floor with weight on the ankles, Japanese style. If a chair is necessary, sit on the corner, free of the back, with feet flat on the floor. If unable to sit on a corner of a seat, sit on a chair with a back but not leaning into it; keep your feet solidly planted on the floor.

b) Stretch the spinal column upward. The term "sit up straight" means that the lower spine, hips, navel, shoulders, ears, and top of the head align with each other.

c) Concentrate the weight and body mass from the shoulders downward at a position two inches below the navel.

d) Pull the chin back and extend the head upward to continue the spinal column line.

e) Relax in this position. Place the tongue behind the upper teeth.

f) Gently close the teeth together into their natural position.

g) Breathe through the nose.

h) Looking straight ahead, relax your gaze and eyelids until they are comfortably half-open or gently closed.

i) Cup the palms of your hands; place the left hand under the right with fingers overlapping as comfortably as possible. The tips of the thumbs may or may not touch. Another position is with the thumb and index finger touching and the back of the hands resting on the knees (mudra).

j) Keeping the spine straight and body relaxed, find the position that minimizes pain and discomfort, even if it is necessary to forgo the lotus or kneeling positions. Investigate, experiment, and find what works for you.

k) Draw the breath quietly through the nose, down to your center, tanden. Try to visualize the circulation of air. The vibrating spiral rhythm of the universe manifests in one cycle of inhalation/exhalation.

Mental preparation:

With this positioning and method of breathing, we now begin meditation. Immediately the mind and physical senses become active. Do not become attached to what appears. Let all thoughts and sensations pass without acting on them.

The highest level of consciousness in budo, Japanese martial arts, is munen muso, meaning "movement without attachment." Buddhist nirvana is munen muso.

If our mind's Qi is stuck on the physical (**U**) or intellectual (**O**) level, the current of Qi will die there. The source of karma is the mind becoming stuck on one thought or sensation. The current must circulate and purify these karma points, **U** and **O**. Misogi halai is the exercise for this purification. Once past the steps of **U** and **O**, the world of **A** will open to you. This is the world existing before the world we see daily. This is the world of gods and Buddhas. From level **A**, we can see and hear beautiful things. Here is the inspiration of artists and the source of religion. It is the sentimental level. Stepping into **E** and **I** takes one deeper and higher, culminating in the Kototama Principle.

This may or may not be easy to understand, but only by sitting and practicing do we come to know the workings of our mind. The practice of sitting meditation and rhythmic breathing can lead to synchronizing with natural life.

People, mountains, sky, sun, moon, stars, water—all these phenomenal world features may help purify and lead one upward. But to follow the most direct path to **IE**, it is necessary to work with a senior student who has traveled the direct path via a senior who has traveled with a senior.

Until now, all spiritual development has led to **A** dimension. Reaching this level of growth has not been too difficult. Prayer, ritual, deprivation, yoga, marijuana, hashish, and psychedelics have provided entrance to this world, but reaching beyond and passing through to **E** to **I** dimensions is far more difficult.

Strong spiritual types arise at the A dimension level, including clairvoyants, prophets, and strong leaders of spiritual groups, societies, and churches. Individuals also dwell at the **A** dimension level, the halfway point of understanding universal life. **A** dimension is the progress the human seed seeks and is the current that flows toward the **I** dimension. Those who have experienced this spiritual space are urged to continue their meditation and practice, not stop the flow.

The biggest mistake the practicant can make is to open the "doors of perception," step through and stop, thinking, "I've got it'" or "I'm home." No, dwelling in the spiritual realm is the beginning of the journey, not the end.

After moving past the place of **A** dimension, one reaches the level/place/space of **E** dimension, or the world of the bodhisattva, or Bosatsu, in Japanese, on the path of exemplifying the four Buddhist virtues. This is the space of perfect natural judgment, the place of the highest morality of human beings.

The last step is that of **I**—the fifty sounds of God. It is known as Kototama, Futomani, manna, Maya (the mother of Buddha), or Logos, the principle that gives birth to Buddha. This is the truth of final human capacity available to all humans. It is said this level of our capacity or knowledge of it has been the spiritual treasure of our ancestors, ever present yet well concealed.

The Three Aspects of Tai Kyoku Practice

Degrees of study and practice vary from simple to intricate, uncomplicated to sophisticated, and relaxed to very intense. The style or system used depends on the way and the practitioner. A practitioner of aikido, a practitioner of meridian therapy, an ill person, a school student, a senior citizen, or a spiritual aspirant will all have unique needs and degrees of investment in these practices. Thus, there are other expressions of the methods: spiritual, mental, medical, martial, and wellness techniques blended, borrowed, and bent concepts and practices to achieve favorable outcomes.

However, though there are many tai kyoku keiko/qigong styles follow the same basic concepts that break down into three aspects. Some schools practice one approach; others use more than one course.

In Kototama Medicine, tai kyoku is the source of power, timing, and form. Through the study of kyoku—breath– that mind and body are united and understood to be the same. In Kototama training, kyoku manifests as forms of misogi – spiritual purification— through breathwork. Sound practice, chanting, and attentive reading are aspects of breathwork. Ego deprivation involves learning to breathe. It is the first step in learning Kototama medicine and spiritual enhancement. Second, kyoku is integral to developing hand Qi, diagnosing, and treating. Third, it is inherent in holding your body as you improve body Qi in stillness and movement. Passing Kototama Life Medicine to the next generation requires concentrated study and understanding of Nakazono Osensei's message and daily usage in experiencing life.

School of Breath Control: Kokyu is breath— the first movement and principle of being. The value begins with developing the mind, breath, and Qi. Development of the universal body and development of the individual body. Kokyu is the bridge between body and soul. Breath is the first and last act of life. It is the most direct method of reconnecting the physical body with the energetic body. Spiritual practitioners, physicians, martial artists, midwives, priests, sages, witches, and shamans have researched the breath for thousands of years, developing and refining breath to address disease, promote relaxation, increase mental focus, and calm the spirit. They used breath to achieve dynamic physical, mental, and spiritual balance, restoring shin Qi (core vitality). Tai Kyoku Keiko eliminates stress, promotes inner tranquility, and aids increased longevity. Inochi style focuses on Kototama sound exercise, physical breath exercise, healing breath exercise, and spiritual development breath exercise.

School of Body Movement and Posture: Physical development in Tai Kyoku Keiko may be highly structured or freeform. Practices may include sitting and standing static postures, undemanding body movements, natural expressions of human and nonhuman actions, or refined martial art forms, such as aikido and tai chi. Inochi style is no force, freeform movement, and structured stretches synchronized with breath and sound, as taught by Nakazono Osensei.

School of Meditation: This approach to increasing the body's energy and balancing the meridians relies on regaining the jurisdiction of the mind. Unique styles may use sound, color, and energy patterns, such as mandalas or five-element guides, to accomplish results. Some meditations are very structured and have specific dictates; some involve focusing on meridians, tsubo, chest movements, or breathing. Some are more exercises in contemplation with a free form or concentrated attention to concepts and ideas. Inochi meditation focuses on breath, sounds, hand Qi exercise, and the Buddhist "one-pointedness of mind' technique. Thousands of years of application by untold millions of practitioners show us the path of skillful development of Qi leads to health, personal growth, and spiritual achievement.

Kototama Five Element Tai Kyoku Practice

A general health practice to stimulate life preservation and expansion through the reproductive, digestive, excretory, and respiratory systems: Labeled *100-day purification* may take up to three months to feel the full benefits. However, most people can feel an immediate improvement in their health, relaxation, adeptness, and mental clarity:

Nakazono misogi purification diet, Kototama spiritual development in breath, movement, and sound meditate focusing on the Kototama Go Gyo: five dimensions of Life Energy expressing the five paired meridians, **A, I, E, O, U** - these are employed to awaken the sacred spaces, Shimpo/Sansho and Ninmyaku/Tokumyaku, termed by Osensei the 'twilight meridians,' where apriori and aposteriori meridians couple. These exercises open, cleanse, heal, and increase energy in these systems.

Nakazono Misogi Purification Diet
Man belongs to the class of animals that eat cereals as the main food, not meat or grasses.

Masahilo M. Nakazono

Nakazono Osensei provided his "Healing Diet" in his textbook, *The Law and Therapy of Natural Life (*© 1978, 1981). Much of the following is from that text.

Do purification diets in the seasons when Life Energy is within yin/yang balance: Spring, the beginning of expansion, and Autumn, the onset of contraction. Summer and winter seasons are extreme, unbalanced, lop-sided, and inappropriate for attempting purification exercises.

Harmony with the environment is absolutely the greatest law for all universal dimensions—the plant and animal worlds or the finite world in general. Not to harmonize is to die.

The Law and Therapy of Natural Life

Cleansing diets may rapidly release congestion, stagnation, and toxins. Therefore, someone who is health deficient should obtain meridian therapy and address dietary adequacies before attempting this way of healing.

The week before the diet begins, if appropriate, decrease the quantity of food per meal.

This purification journey ends where it begins. Therefore, if you need to finish the process early, try to "back out of it," reverse the time and menu you have already partaken.

As a body/mind/spirit purification process, avoid stressful situations, intense exercise, extreme temperature changes, and drafts. Be mindful. This exercise is a minimum of 5260 days in length.

The principal food consists of whole grains: amaranth, barley, buckwheat, corn, millet, oats, quinoa, rice, rye, and wheat. It is best to eat grain whole, but if cracked or ground, consume it within that week. Whole brown rice is a powerful essential food for healing. Try them all.

The side dishes may be dried vegetables, leafy vegetables, root vegetables, sea vegetables, and legumes. [Osensei stated the energies of eggplant, (white) potatoes, and tomatoes are "too strongly expansive" and not used in a cleansing diet.]

Sauté the vegetables in a lightly oiled (sesame) pan and add water and steam. When nearly done, you may add sea salt, natural miso, tamari, or soy sauce to taste. Taste and cooking length must be harmonious with health issues and symptoms.

Pre-First Step:

Days One through Fourteen: a moderate three-meal exercise. Eat whole grains, lightly cooked vegetables, miso soup, fish or tofu, green tea, and umeboshi plum. Chew slowly, carefully, and consciously. Slowly drink a glass (8 oz) of filtered water between each meal.

First Step:

Days Fifteen through Twenty: two meals a day.

<u>Main dish</u>: one bowl of cooked brown rice with one teaspoonful of gomashio [gently ground, toasted sesame seed (80 percent), blended with toasted sea salt (20 percent)].

Cook grains a little firm.

"When it is too soft, you do not chew it well enough, and you swallow it too soon. This is the wrong way to eat because not enough saliva is produced, which is an essential part of digestion. Cook one cup of rice with 1½ cups of water. Start with low heat and raise it as the water heats up. After it starts to bubble, lower the heat again. Cover the pot with a tight, heavy lid to avoid losing any liquid. Keep on low heat for about 30 minutes. Pressure cooking is all right but follows the same principle.
Steam is essential; let the pot sit covered after it has cooked.

Masahilo M Nakazono
The Law and Therapy of Natural Life

Use chopsticks, a fork, or a spoon to obtain a mouthful (120130 grains) of rice/gomashio. Chew each mouthful until it slides down without effort, uninduced swallowing: "Drink your solids."

Side dishes:

a. Sautéed vegetables. One tablespoonful at each meal.
b. Miso soup cooked with sea vegetables, root crops, or leaf vegetables. Half a rice bowl full, once a day.
c. A small amount of the meat of white fish, freshwater fish, or tiny fish that are eaten whole may be added to the miso soup for flavor, especially when cold; however, it is not necessary. Tofu is excellent; the heat of the cooked miso modifies its yin abundance.
d. One umeboshi plum with each meal.

Fluids:

a) Natural, filtered water, about eight ounces between each meal per day.

b) Freshly squeezed vegetable juice, one 6-ounce cup per day

c) "Distinctive brews": barley tea, brown rice tea, brown rice bancha tea, vegetable broth; 2-3 teacups a day

Drink fluids slowly and mix well with saliva in your mouth before allowing it to slide down your throat. Do not swallow. 'Eat your liquids.'

Make all juices and brews fresh and drink immediately after preparation. If not practical, juice only enough for the day and store in the refrigerator in a closed container. Vegetables should be at room temperature before juicing; juices should be at room temperature before consumption.

Rubbing Therapy:

Rub your body daily using a dry cloth or a tawashi (Japanese scrubbing brush) and rub until your whole body has warmed up. Rub your body with your hand where you feel stiffness or pain, slightly press there for a short while; rub your entire body with a towel dampened with icy water and wrung out or take an alternating hot and cold shower. Force nothing.

Shower Therapy:

While showering, alternate hot and cold water, thirty seconds hot and thirty seconds cold. Once habituated, lengthen to one minute each and end with cold water. While showering, vigorously rub with a towel or tawashi brush until the skin is red.

Exercise:

Use movement exercises found in this book. Once in the morning and once in the afternoon, your strength and condition set the tone. Force nothing.

Elimination:

Average urinating frequency is three to five times a day, about every five to eight hours. If the frequency is above average, you are drinking too much liquid, or it is symptomatic of a disorder. If the frequency is below average, suspect it is a symptom. When urine quantity is minimal, it may be that kidney-bladder meridians are yin jitsu/yang kyo or the person is over-perspiring; if it is above average, suspect yin kyo/yang jitsu.

The standard color of urine is light yellow. If it is a very thick yellow or brownish, suspect an inner fever. If it is white, suspect a sodium deficiency or diabetes.

Bowel evacuations usually occur daily; more than three times is not ordinary. The stools are brown to slightly brownish yellow, neither hard nor soft, with no unpleasant smell. A light-yellow color or too soft or too hard (constipated) is not standard.

Some people may already react to this first step of the regime and be unable to continue to the next step. In such a situation, you may continue the first step but not longer than one month. If this step is to extend more than one month, the guidance of a specialist is desirable. The first step is usually enough to heal a light sickness.

Second Step:

Days Twenty-One through Twenty-Four:

Main dish: 70 percent whole rice porridge; one rice bowl twice a day.

70 Percent Porridge: Cook 1 cup rice (grain) to 10 cups water, wellcovered on low heat for about 2 hours, reducing the liquid by 30 percent, then turn off the heat and let it sit. When it has cooled, squeeze through a cheesecloth. Discard the liquid.

Side dish: Same as Step One but in smaller amounts. One umeboshi plum per meal. Eat the second meal before sunset.

Fluids: Same as in Step One. Note the condition of the urine. If it is too much or too frequent, reduce the amount of liquid consumed.

Days Twenty-Five and Twenty-Six:

Main dish: 50 percent liquid reduction whole rice porridge; one rice bowl twice daily.

Side dish: None, except one umeboshi plum per meal.

Fluids: Same as in First Step. Observe the condition of the urine.

3) Days Twenty-Seven & Twenty-Eight:

Main dish: 30 percent whole rice porridge (70 percent liquid reduction); one rice bowl, twice a day.

Side dish: None, except one umeboshi plum per meal. Fluids: Same as in First Step. Pay attention to urine.

4) Day Twenty-Nine:

Main dish: Rice soup, only the liquid from the 30 percent cooked rice; one rice bowl, twice a day.
Side dish: None, except one umeboshi plum per meal.

Fluids: Same as in First Step. Pay attention to urine.
Do not drink more than two cups of additional liquid daily; watch the amount of urine and adjust your fluids accordingly. Try to continue with exercise and massage according to each person's condition and strength; do not force it.

Third Step:

Four: Days Thirty through Thirty-Four:

This is a fasting phase: Fluids are the same as in the first step. Employ movement exercises found in this book, once in the morning and once in the afternoon, depending on your strength and condition.

Fourth Step:

Day Thirty-Five:

<u>Main dish:</u> Whole rice soup; one bowl, twice a day.

<u>Side dish:</u> One umeboshi plum per meal.

<u>Fluids:</u> Same as in First Step.

    1) Days Thirty-Six and Thirty-Seven:

        <u>Main dish:</u> 30 percent whole rice porridge; one bowl twice daily.

        <u>Side dish:</u> umeboshi plum per meal

        <u>Fluids:</u> Same as in First Step.

    2) Days Thirty-Eight through Forty:
        <u>Main dish:</u> 50 percent whole rice porridge; one bowl twice daily.

        <u>Side dish:</u> One umeboshi plum per meal.

        <u>Fluids:</u> Same as in First Step.

Days Forty-One through Forty-Five:

Main dish: 70 percent whole rice porridge; one bowl twice daily.

Side dish: One umeboshi plum per meal.

Fluids: Same as in First Step.

Fifth Step:

1) Return to the First Step for a week to ten days; then, you may return to normal eating.

During this diet, you should very carefully monitor the patient's condition, noting emotional, mental, physical (**A/O/U**) strength, and if there are any changes. If, at any point, you sense something profound in their condition, stop there. Take your patient back slowly through the previous steps, in reverse order, until they are back to normal eating. To go suddenly from the second or third step back to normal eating could be problematic, so be careful not to do this. On the return, when your patient starts eating again, they usually feel ravenous and want to eat a lot. Be especially careful at that time! That mistake can destroy the whole effect of the diet and cause the patient to develop a more severe condition.

The practitioner must continually carefully monitor the patient, correctly diagnosing the condition. The most critical point of diet therapy is deciding when to go ahead or when to go back, taking the steps very slowly. Do not forget this! Fluids and exercise may be increased or reduced per the patient's strength. The practitioner needs to have enough experience to judge correctly. Do not be so ridiculous as to think that observing counts as experience; do not be so dangerous to society as to think, "I got it!"

CHAPTER SEVEN

BREATHING

Breath Kappo

Breath is the first act of individual life; we inhale at birth.
Breath is the last act of individual life; we exhale at death.

SELF-HEALTH

Self-healthcare practices are rooted in the past, but their need could be no greater than our present time. The high anxiety of modern living, geopolitical unrest, shifts in our ecosystem, and our immune systems require practices that strengthen the mind/body/spirit, enhance the serenity of the heart, and benefit the entire system. The exercise involves the communion of body/mind/spirit. When doing self-care handwork, go slowly; this is also true when providing therapy to others. Do not overwork a sick person, including yourself; perform gentle exercises. These self-purification exercises are for use for the rest of your life. First, master them; when understood, they are yours; then, you can instruct others in self-healthcare. What is yours, you may share.

Self-Health Starts With the Breath

"Iki: I–Life ki–qi. IKI is the Breath of Life, that is, the Qi of Life-Will; the 'unborn' Qi, from which universal and individual breath begins. Iki is the Source breath, the Breath before Breath. Kyoku is breath, the first movement, the First Principle of Being. This is not an abstract thought. The First Principle begins with the flow of mind, Breath, and Qi, the Universal body's movement, and the individual body's movement. Kyoku, breath, is the bridge between body and soul."

Masahilo M. Nakazono, class notes

Most people in the United States live fearful, stressful lives and have shallow breathing patterns. When a natural birth occurs, that is, a nontraumatic transition from womb to room, that child will take its first inhalation deep from the lower belly, the tanden. This space, below the umbilicus, is where we naturally breathe. Pain or fear at birth or sometime after results in breathing up in the diaphragm or, worse, the chest, which leads to shortness of breath and inadequate oxygen supply to the brain and body, resulting in anxiety and hypofunction. A human born nonviolently takes its first breath deep in the lower belly, an easily verifiable universal truth. Breathing into and out from the tanden is the design. You think I am repeating myself; you are still breathing shallow.

I have had the privilege of attending natural births. I am referring to births that are vaginal without interference. No drugs, surgeries, no instruments like forceps, no invasive activities. Just natural, healthy, nonmedical actuality that over 98 percent of birthing mothers worldwide experience without incidence. Only 75 years ago, modern medicine grasped the financial benefit of treating pregnancy as a health issue and insisted that births occur in disease-centric hospitals. My mother was born at home. Most of my children were born at home. I was born in a hospital. I am here to report that much is lost with hospital births, starting with the first breath.

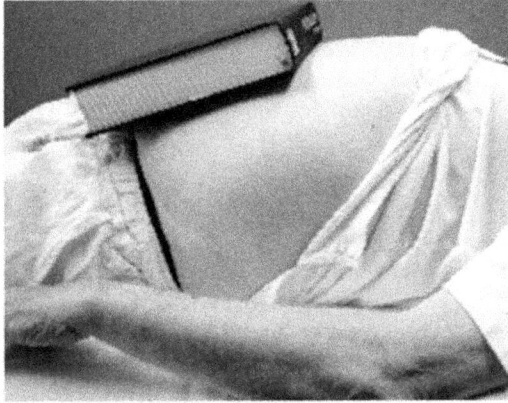

The Practice

An exercise for retraining and regaining tanden breathing is to lie on your back on a firm surface and place a heavy book, some counterweight, on tanden, located the width of three fingers below the umbilicus. Practice inhaling that causes the lower abdomen to rise at tanden, pushing the counterweight upward.

Alternatively, instead of a counterweight, have a person place a hand there and maintain firm pressure. Effecting with a partner allows two people to study adequate breathing and allows your partner to help you remember not to hyperventilate during the practice. Your partner can monitor your breathing and guide you from breathing too rapidly. You can reverse roles, and both can experience healing breaths and the physiological reconnection to your original moment of independent life, the breath at birth.

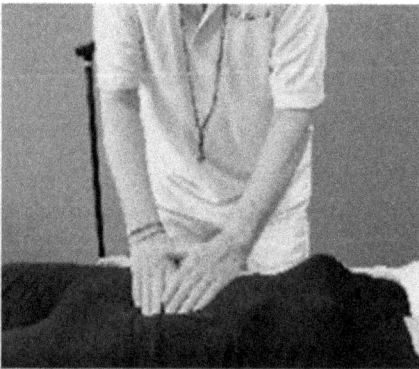

Practice alone or with another, but practice at least five minutes daily. Then, as tanden breathing becomes more familiar and comfortable, begin attending to tanden breathing in all positions and always: sitting, standing, walking, driving, and talking and still breathing from tanden, always returning to tanden. Keep practicing this way until it becomes second nature, a weird phrase because you want this to become first nature. Work to regain what you lost around the time of your birth.

Once you have begun the practice of reconnecting with tanden, you can start disciplined breathing exercises as medicine. Pain will transform, and problems will disappear with deep breathing. This is the first step toward regaining health.

Many books teach many ways, old and new, of breath exercise. Most are repeats or rebranding of one another; there are ancient practices with new names or new techniques claiming to be ancient. Study them all if you want but keep breathing while studying.

In addition to Kototama Fifty Sounds practice (below), Nakazono Osensei provided three Shugendo breath exercises:

1. Healing Breath
2. Development of Spirit Breath
3. Inner Discrimination Breath This third exercise is not a treatment; it is solely for developing inner judgment to achieve rhythm with **IE**, Life-Will/Life-Power.

Nakazono Osensei believed all levels of healing, accomplished through breath exercises, could be achieved through the Kototama Fifty Sounds. I suggest you attempt to master each phase of these three exercises while continuing Kototama sound practice. (described below)

Begin breathing exercises in the morning. Guide yourself to deep breathing, into and out of tanden, the Sea of Qi. This will revitalize energy.

Even for one who is extremely sick or old, deep breathing exercises (healing breath #1) may revitalize Life Energy. On the "death bed," deep breathing can seem like a miracle, but it is not; it is merely the reawakening of Qi.

Place your hand on the lower abdomen.
Breathe.

Breathe in through the nose, sensing the Qi force flowing over your head, down your back, and into the Sea of Qi, tanden, the center of your physical and spiritual being, two inches below your navel. Exhale through your mouth, sensing Qi flowing from your tanden, up the front of your body, and out. Breathe thoroughly and slowly so that there is no sound. Practice breathing in tanden. Keep your spine straight, as if hanging from a cord attached to the crown of your head.

Morning is the best time to practice these exercises, although, throughout the day, you should continuously breathe deeply into your lower abdomen. Never breathe only in your chest.

Practice until mastered, and then instruct family and friends, patients, and everyone. There are three levels or phases of practice and proficiency. Start with the primary stage and progress only as you become at home with each step.

Healing Breath

(Normal breath patterns for ordinary people under normal circumstances)

The first moment and movement of teate is in the breath. These self-purification exercises are for your use for the rest of your life. First, master these exercises. In this way, you will be able to instruct others in self-healthcare. This first breath exercise can be beneficial for ill people; even extremely sick people can be helped quite powerfully. For sick or weak people, you must support their breathing by placing your hand on their tanden; as they strengthen, guide them to doing it alone.

First Phase: There are six complete breaths in one minute. Inhale for 5 seconds. Exhale for 5 seconds.

 Second Phase: There are four complete breaths in one minute. Inhale for 7 seconds. Exhale for 7 seconds.

Third Phase: There are three complete breaths in one minute. Inhale for 10 seconds. Exhale for 10 seconds.

As you practice this breath pattern, observe its effects on your mood and health. Perhaps keep a journal.

Development of Spirit Breath

(Healing breath pattern to develop physical and spiritual capacity in a healthy person).

Development of Spirit Breath is for spiritual practices, healing, calming practices, and, most significantly, self-healing. Incorporate into all your exercises. After it is yours, you may share it with like-minded people, parallel travelers on the narrow path.

First Phase: There are four complete breaths in one minute. Inhale for 5 seconds. Hold for 5 seconds. Exhale for 5 seconds.

Second Phase: There are 2.86 breath cycles per minute. Inhale for 7 seconds. Hold breath for 7 seconds. Exhale for 7 seconds.

 Third Phase: There are two complete breaths in one minute. Inhale for 10 seconds. Hold breath for 10 seconds. Exhale for 10 seconds.

Inner Discrimination Breath   (Breath of Judgment)
(Spiritual breath patterns for the initiate, NOT for treatment purposes)

This breath pattern exercise is solely for developing inner judgment to achieve rhythm with *IE*, Life-Will/Life-Power. It needs to be practiced and mastered within the context and practice of your spiritual studies, and it is most powerful with the studies and exercises of Kototama Sound.

First Phase: There are two complete breaths per minute. Inhale for 7 seconds, hold breath for 7 seconds, exhale for 7 seconds, hold breath for 7 seconds, inhale for 7 seconds, hold the breath for 7 seconds, exhale for 7 seconds, hold the breath for 7 seconds. Continue.

Second Phase: There are one and a half cycles each minute. Inhale for 10 seconds, hold the breath for 10 seconds, exhale for 10 seconds, hold for 10 seconds, inhale for 10 seconds. Continue.

Third Phase: There is one breath per minute. Inhale for 15 seconds, hold your breath for 15 seconds, exhale for 15 seconds, hold for 15 seconds. Continue.

In these studies, do not use the mind as a thinking device; become aware of the cerebral vibration, the energy behind thought, the sum of the brain.

KOTOTAMA SOUND THERAPY:
AWAKEN TANDEN WITH THE SOUND
RHYTHM OF SU A WA

A useful practice is to inhale into tanden, exhale, forming the audible sound **SU**; repeat fifty **SU**s per session as a daily exercise. This is natural self-healthcare; work on it. Be patient; you have twenty or more years of damage to repair.

This way of breathing provides oxygen to our entire being. Our spiritual self, our decisive self, our intentional self, our mental self, and our physical self all benefit.

"Practice begins with the pronunciation of the sounds aloud. When meditating, breathe slowly and extend each breath as long as possible. Breathe deeply through the tanden, not the chest.

"Begin with the sound SU, then A-WA. Do not use any technique or embellishment, such as a melody. Let the sounds come out naturally; otherwise, you are beginning with intellectual activity and will not be able to see anymore.

"To make sounds is an action of expansion. It should start from the point of final concentration, the absolute center. Always start with the teeth firmly together.

"The rhythm of sounds, our life's manifestation, is based on (I) dimension, Life Will. When making the (I) sounds, the teeth remain closed by biting the teeth.

"A-E-O-U, the four dimensions of mother sounds, and the child sounds come out from (I). With each sound, always return to biting the teeth.

*"**A** sound is energy expanding to the fullest and formed with a fully opened mouth.*

*"Make the **O** with a round mouth, half-closed; the tiniest opening comes out as **U** sound.*

*"**I** and **E** sounds, with the mouth open sideways. The teeth open for the **E** sound but remain closed for the **I** sound. The same inner energy is expanding, only the form of the mouth changes. Our human Life Energy expands in only these five ways—these five sounds.*

*"When making the **WA** sounds, sound it out as **U-U-U-WA**; you can see it better that way. Try to realize the difference between the light of **A** and **WA**. No shrine or ceremony uses only one candle. There are always two lights which symbolize the manifestation of human capacity and **A** and **WA**."* Inochi, The Book of Life

Vowel sounds as a developmental breath technique:

Make each sound for as long as possible in one breath and with a full voice.

A: the mouth is fully open, large, and round

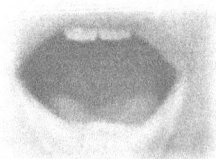

I: bite the teeth, opening the lips sideways.

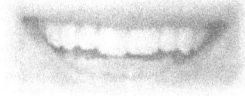

E: from the I-position, open the teeth.

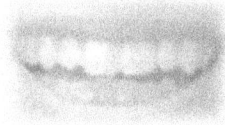

O: open the mouth halfway, making it round.

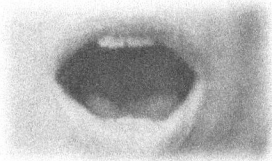

U: make the mouth small and round.

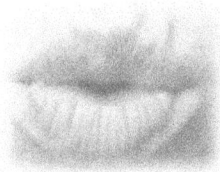

Do this exercise, breathing deeply and with the most in- depth concentration of spirit. It may be executed sitting, lying down, or standing; the body should be naturally erect, the spine, fluid. Sound out from the tanden, located a few inches below the navel.

One performs breathing exercises by expressing pure human sound, A I E O U. Vowel sounds are the same in nearly all languages, the root sound in every word, the "soul" of the word. Vowel sounds are a form of contemplation, meditation, and prayer to purify speech, not only my speech but also the word sounds coming out of everyone's mouth. Listen to them.

Vowel sounds as a breathing and diagnostic technique:
A (ah) Spirit, Emotion, Awakening, Growth
E (a) Judgment, Decisive, Affirmation, Inhalation
I (ee) Will, Intent, Expression, Motivation
O (o) Mind, Psychic, Mental, Thought, Memory, Continuity
U (oo) Body, Form, Physical, Nourishment

Sounds to be read from top to bottom and right to left.

SUGASO

WA	NA	LA	MA	YA	HA	SA	KA	TA .	A
WO	NO	LO	MO	YO	HO	SO	KO	TO	O
WU	NU	LU	MU	YU	HU	SU	KU	TU	U
WE	NE	LE	ME	YE	HE	SE	KE	TE	E
WI	NI	LI	MI	YI	HI	SI	KI.	TI	I

KANAGI

WA LA YA MA HA NA TA SA KA A
WI LI YI MI HI NI TI SI KI   I
WU LU YU MU HU NU TU SU KU   U
WE LE YE ME HE NE TE SE KE E
WO LO YO MO HO NO TO SO KO O

FUTONORITO

WA SA YA NA LA HA MA KA TA   A
WI SI YI NI LI HI MI KI TI   I
WE SE YE NE LE HE ME KE TE   E
WO SO YO NO LO HO MO KO TO O
WU SU YU NU LU HU MU KU TU U

Use the vowel sounds as a breathing technique, as a form of contemplation, meditation, and prayer; use to purify speech, mind, and everyone. This way of breathing provides oxygen to our entire being, our spiritual self, our judgment capacity, our will to live, our mental awareness, and our physical body.

CHAPTER EIGHT

HAND SPIRIT QI TEATE

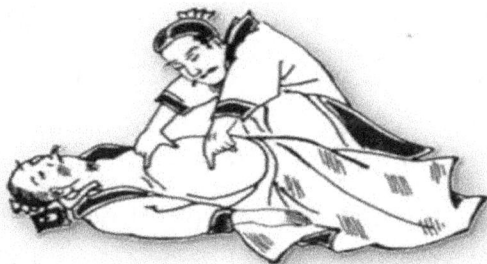

When treating, use everything you can: acupuncture, handwork, moxibustion, diet, electricity, herbs, meditation, exercise, laser, psychology, psychiatry, philosophy, nutrition, shock therapy, humor, spiritual activity, meditation, and deprivation. You draw on everything. You must know the dosage— how much and when. This is the natural physician's work.

INOCHI TAI QI TEATE

Treatment includes Sakai Hon Rei Teate, Nakazono-style ampuku (abdominal massage) and kappo, Kototama breathwork and sound therapy, anma, shiatsu, hari (acupuncture), kyu (moxibustion), and kampo (herbal medicine).

Anma, traditional Japanese massage, encompasses many techniques, including light to medium finger pressure gently applied to move or stimulate the muscles by pressing, kneading, and rubbing. Muscles are never "rolled;" kneading is what they need, like making bread, but gently, invigorating the body's energy. Sedate overexcited nerves and muscles by pressing (an), sha/liberate. Deterioration in the functional integrity of physical systems requires rubbing (ma), ho/enhance.

Shiatsu, traditional Japanese soft-tissue manipulation by hands, fingers, thumbs, elbows, and feet, intentionally influences the flow of meridian energy (Qi). The primary meridians, extraordinary meridians, and Go Gyo regions of the body receive this therapy. With anma and shiatsu, practitioners use thumbs, individual fingers, feet, knees, and elbows to achieve the proper stimulation. Some practitioners use a technique that employs a porcelain rice spoon to rub the skin. We do not need that; it seems too violent. It is more natural to massage with your hands and feel the response. Treatment is in touch, not the tool. This is especially true when employing a tool.

Shiatsu and anma are useful for treating soft tissue injuries. They are used to relax tendons, stimulate meridians, relieve cramps and spasms, relieve pain, promote the circulation of Qi, blood, and lymph, accelerate metabolism, address stagnation (obstruction), which reduces edema (swelling), and resolves fascial and muscular adhesions.

Ampuku ("calm the abdomen"), a traditional Japanese abdominal diagnosis and treatment method used in Go Gyo meridian therapy; ju and shaku (deep and superficial Qi and blood stagnation) treatment; fukushin diagnosis and kampo therapy; and tactile therapies, such as shiatsu and abdominal massage. Sakai Sensei's comprehensive treatment method is essential in our studies and procedures relating to abdominal therapy. Helpful for your studies and your patients. When you are ready to seek what Sakai Sensei sought, let go of all thoughts or ideas and let your hand Qi harmonize with the Qi of your partners' abdomen. Experience nothing.

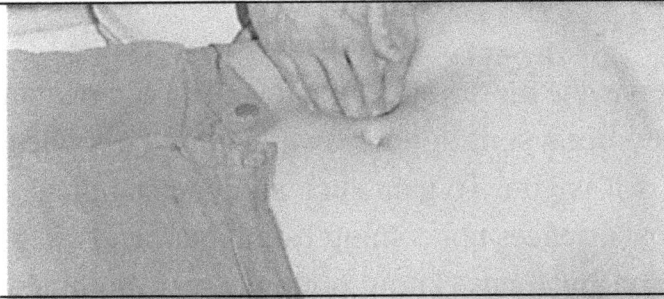

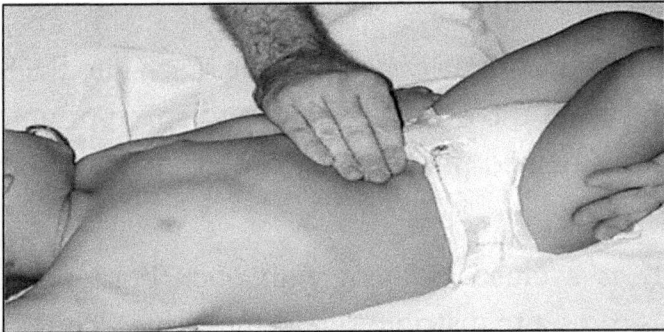

Kappo ("taking back" or "correcting mistakes") is traditional resuscitation therapy developed primarily through martial arts. The development of martial arts necessitated developing ways of fixing what was being broken. Thus, trauma medicine always makes advances because of war-type activity. In the old days, many advanced healing arts practitioners were also masters of the martial arts, including Masahilo M. Nakazono, who was highly ranked in aikido, kendo, karate, and judo. Traditional practitioners in East Asia studied how to correct dysfunction of soft, skeletal, and connective tissue while attending to the internal organs and senses and the emotional and spiritual components within the dysfunction. They applied soaks, salves, plasters, compresses, acupuncture, moxibustion, herbal medicines, massage, manipulative therapies, stretches, movement, exercises, and diet. In addition, they taught centering, meditation, quieting the mind, stress management, self- healthcare, and cooking, passing on to us all the manual therapies, movement, exercises, empirical wisdom, and spiritual wisdom that arose through the healing arts and martial arts.

The more you receive, the more you retain; the more you maintain, the more you know because it is your own acquired knowledge. "It's yours," means it is you. To gain such an understanding, one must let go of all experiences not coming from your hands. This is part of what I mean by focus: know nothing, seek nothing, do nothing; gain attentiveness to energy.

We energize our hands, becoming conscious; we reach into the Sea of Qi and sound out from the original sound and space of union, the first-born place of named phenomena, center; and we sound out SU.

> The body is a closed system with open borders. Life Energy is present; distribution is the issue. Thus, we experience through diagnosis and treatment that if there is a deficiency (kyo) condition in the system, there is also an excess (jitsu) state. Our task is to equalize, get back to the center, bring back into focus, and bring back into synchronization situations of unbalance. When you take pulses, you are looking for this. When you do teate, you are attempting to address this. With hari, you must be exact in your diagnosis and subsequent treatment. You may injure by putting a needle in the wrong meridian and

compromise the healing experience by planting it in the wrong point or wrong direction.

Nakazono Osensei, certified in kappo in 1938, trained his students in manipulative

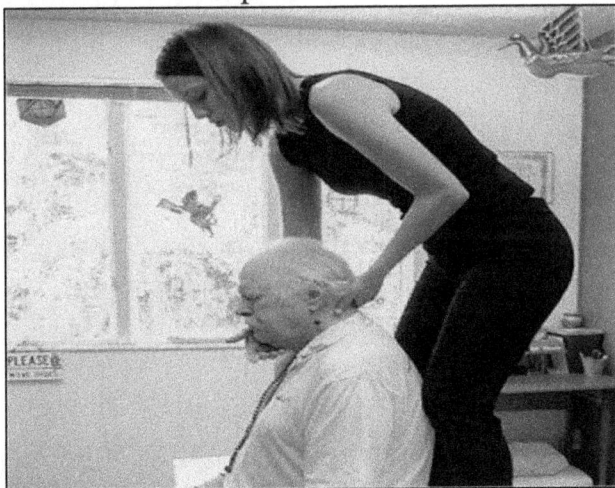

therapies and various "take-back" techniques of the traditional kappo practitioner. Such techniques aid in vital Qi reawakening, meridian patency, postural alignment, and support of deeper and subtler aspects of the body's organs, spirit, and function. Advanced first aid, emergency medical techniques, and cardiopulmonary resuscitation are examples of modern kappo techniques. Physical therapy, occupational therapy, massage therapy, chiropractic therapy, and structural integration (Rolfing) are potentially in the realm of kappo; it depends on the intent and capacity of the practitioner. Before I studied traditional medicine, I trained as an emergency medical technician. I encourage students and practitioners of traditional medicine to take advanced first aid or EMT courses as part of their primary studies. I have also encouraged students and practitioners of contemporary (modern) medicine to take advanced first aid or EMT courses.

Sotai is simple movements to restore and maintain balance. When the body is imbalanced or distorted for any reason, the center of gravity will shift. It may be a slight shift, but it will cause the center of mass to move. Bodyworkers see this all the time. For example, a slightly curved spine, one shoulder higher than the other, and hips or pelvis tilted, even slightly, results in an abnormal gait. These distortions can be problematic and lead to diseases and crippling disorders. This perception is the basis from which sotai developed and operates.

One of the key elements of Dr. Hashimoto's sotai technique is the integration of breath and movement, as in aikido, acupuncture, and shiatsu techniques. All these systems recognize and utilize breath and movement. A "master" of aikido or meridian therapy is a master of their breath.

Dr. Hashimoto, a medical doctor and a physiologist, also drew on previous models that came from East Asia— yoga, anma, shiatsu, and jujitsu. Yoga is a bilateral movement and alignment method that guides the body back into a state of balance or center. Anma showed him how to use "push/pull" techniques to assist the musculature in relaxing; shiatsu showed him the way of pressure and the use of tsubo to affect the desired results of muscular and tendon alignment, and jujitsu provided the centuries-old techniques of kappo. Sotai, a developed form of physical therapy only a few decades old, invented and developed by a Western doctor, falls within the realm of kappo.Teate ("hand/spirit treatment," "hand healing spirit," or "spiritual handwork") is the tactile therapy of Nakazono Osensei and Sakai Sensei, who taught the development of healing Qi in the hands through focused hand-breath-and centeredness. The techniques include

Light rubbing, with fingers straight, palm and fingers flat. Soft kneading, muscle massage with a firm grip.

Squeezing and kneading, with one or two fingers or thumb applying vertical or circular pressure for bones, joints, tendons, and ligaments.

Pressure, micro-touch on the body's surface—not deep muscle tissue— using the hand or thumb with a powerful effect (adjust pressure with the patient's exhalation).

Tapping, with a side of the fist, knuckles, or soft fist to treat the nervous system.

Vibration, with a flat hand for muscles and peripheral nervous system. Sakai Sensei taught and guided Nakazono Osensei in Sakai Hon Rei Teate, and Nakazono Osensei taught and engaged me for many years, as have I with my senior students. Sakai Sensei treated all conditions through abdominal handwork. His way of removing stagnation from the center of life, the abdomen, involves training the hands to express the Qi from the tanden. Hon Rei Teate ("original principle of spiritual handwork") is the abdominal diagnosis and treatment by touch. Sakai Sensei did not take pulses and used no traditional diagnostic techniques. Instead, he provided Qi flowing from tanden through the palms to unite with the stagnations encountered in the abdomen without thought or idea of organs, systems, meridians, goals, or anything other than Qi of hands expressing the Qi of tanden. The intent is quite essential; you must focus on the intention of touching the abdomen; no thought, just purposeless purpose.

As Osensei pointed out, "Teate is art, not science. It is an expression of yourself experiencing yourself. Proficiency will come, but you cannot make it happen.
Mastery is not static; it is moving, evolving, but the underneath spirit remains the same." He invited his students to express themselves in such a way that "if an ancestor came along and

observed what you are mastering, the ancestor would say, 'I have never seen it like this, but it is Teate."

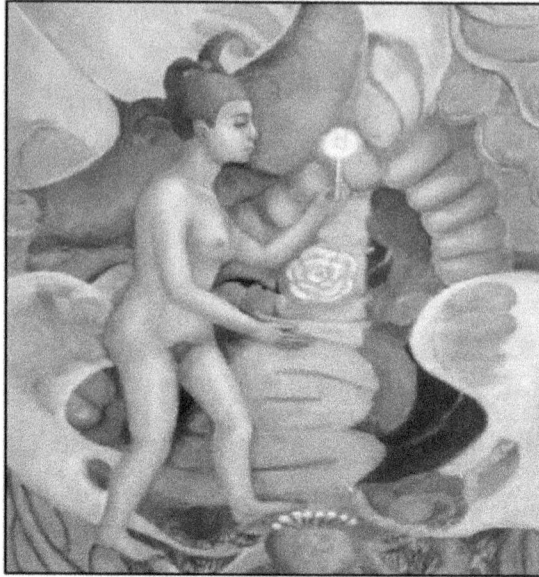

SeekingSelf Knowledge by Monica

KOTOTAMA INOCHI TEATE

The studies begin with hand Qi exercise, accessing tanden through the hands. The union of mind-body-spirit through focused attention to breathing and Qi, as exemplified in the discoveries of Ueshiba Osensei, the Hon Rei Teate teachings of Sakai Sensei, and the work of Masahilo M. Nakazono Osensei. Hand Qi exercise is the center of our meditation, somatic therapy, moxibustion, and acupuncture studies. First, master these exercises, then you can instruct your clientele in self-healthcare. With self-work, you must go slow. These are self-purification exercises to use for the rest of your life and to rest the use of your life.

You should not over-exert if you are ill; do gentle exercises. And, of course, do not overwork the sick person. Not enough is ALWAYS better than too much.

Always start with the intent not to represent your ego. Treating yourself or treating others, treat the same. Be non-judgmental and unattached, with the attitude, *"I do not care as to the outcome; I will just do my very best."* (Nakazono Osensei's mantra, [aka], Karma Yoga)

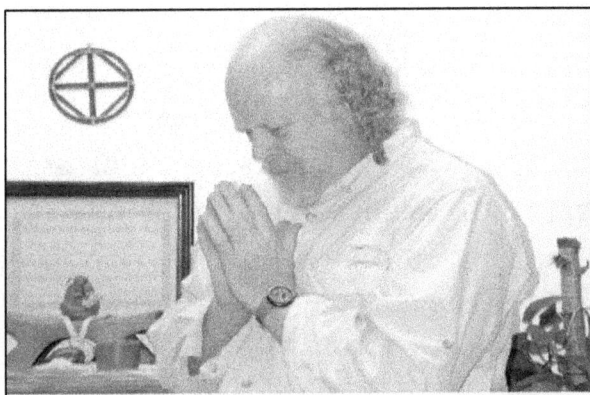

Hand QiExercise

Awakening the "energy body" - the vital life force - *IE* dimension

Spirit healing is not an esoteric concept nor a spiritual phenomenon available only to the initiate, nor is it of religion or casual bodies. Each one of us is living and manifests Life Energy. We are studying the energy of the form and the conscious tapping into Life Energy through deliberate actions of the form itself.

The Sea of Qi is accessed by a centering technique of the hands, the Sakai hand Qi exercise, in which Qi is focused in the epicenter of the hands, separating the hands while Qi is flowing between them until the heat and vibration sense everything. Seventy percent of hand treatment is touching diagnosis.

To access tanden Qi through the hands, one must first gain access to tanden through the breath. Locate the tanden below the navel at Ninmyaku/CV 5 (Sekimon). The Lower Burner (Jo Sho), Ninmyaku/CV 3 (Chukyoku), Ninmyaku/CV 4 (Kangen), Ninmyaku/CV 5 (Sekimon), and
Ninmyaku/CV 6 (Kikai)] can be considered the space of tanden. For our studies, the reference point is about three fingers below the navel. The exact location is the hollow felt with the finger reaching from the tanden.

This hand Qi exercise from Sakai Sensei is fundamental in providing spiritual and physical healthcare. Initially, practice this exercise sitting or kneeling. Your head, shoulders, and hips are aligned and relaxed; the palms of the hands align, and the fingers touch softly. Position your hands as in prayer and focus on the hollow space between your palms as you breathe from tanden. You may feel heat, a sensation, vibration, or magnetism between your hands. This is Qi. Hang out with it. Feel your energy. Allow your hands to separate while continuing to experience the energy flowing between your hands. Spend time practicing this way and experience Qi. When you can feel this energy whenever you bring your palms near each other, you will be near the start of the beginning of the long embryonic journey toward the infancy of energy healing. You cannot quicken this process; you can slow it. One must practice hand Qi every day for ten to thirty minutes.

There is a proverb from Zen or Gestalt Therapy or common sense: "You can't push the river." Do not try to make things happen; partake in the happening. Do not go against the grain.

Gentle is good. Calm is necessary. Take a breath into your tanden; let it out through the sound, SUUUUUUUUUU.

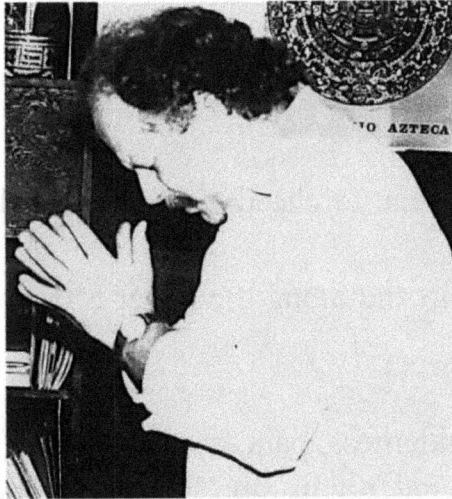

The beginning place of diagnosis and treatment

Self-Handwork

The aspects of hand treatment are Qi, rhythm, and quiet. Develop a balanced combination.

1) Head

Using your fingers, rub down the front of your face, the middle finger down the center of the face.

Rub and press down the center of the head

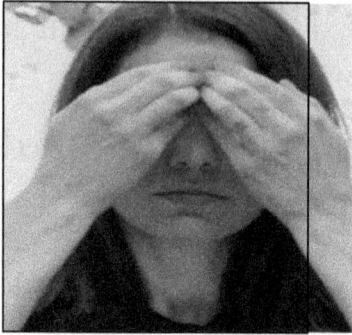

with four fingers: from the forehead to the point below the skull, Tokumyaku #15 (Amon). Then, press up and along the lower Sho Yo Myaku with all five fingers.

Feel for sensitivity, tenderness, pain, hardness—any abnormality. Two beneficial, essential points are lower Sho Yo (GB) #20 (Fuchi) for flu, sinus, and eye issues and lower Sho Yo (GB) #12 (Kankotsu) for mastoid sinus, ear, and inner ear issues. Lower Tai Yo (Bl) #10 (Tenchu) is just to the side of the occipital protuberance.

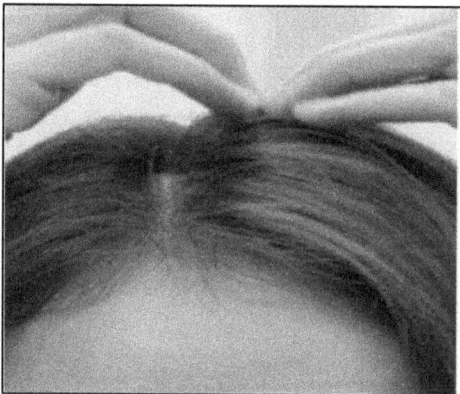

Many conditions are associated with this tsubo (eye problems, nasal problems, heart problems, blood circulation problems, cerebral difficulties, mental problems, head problems, insomnia). Often, tenderness is on the lower Sho Yo myaku tsubo. Use fingertips and push in and upwards under the skull, feeling for hardness, softness, pain, or tenderness. Rub the scalp with your fingers using general overall firm pressure. The idea is to keep the muscles relaxed and the blood, nerve, lymph, and myaku (meridians) open. Address fevers by relieving the pressure exerted on the small blood vessels.

Influencing the elasticity of the blood vessels is vital. This handwork treatment is suitable for high blood pressure; headaches, migraine headaches; abnormal blood circulation in the head; dizziness; blood circulation problems; stiff neck; flu; and sinus issues. Rubbing the head is influential. Rub behind and under the ears. Are there hard contractions? Is there ringing in the ears? Is there elasticity? Lack of flexibility of the flesh of the external ear may indicate deeper problems.

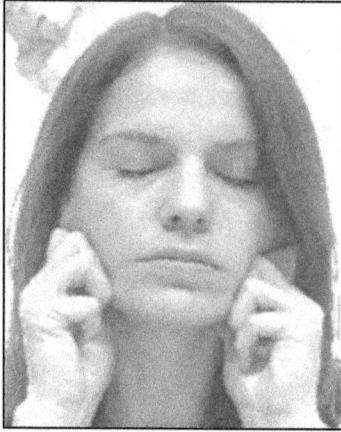

2) Jaw

Press your thumb under and into the jaw from the chin and along the jawbone line, back to the junction under the ears at upper Sho Yo (TH) #17 (Eifu). This is the connecting space of the upper Sho Yo (TH) myaku and lower Sho Yo (GB) myaku. Then press back along the base of the skull to the mastoid process at lower Sho Yo (GB) #12 (Honshin). At the same time, influence the front of the jaw with the thumbs at lower Yo Mei (St) #5 (Daigei), lower Yo Mei (St) #6 (Kyosha), lower Yo Mei (St) #7 (Gekan); these tsubo relate to the gums, teeth, and nerves. Lower Yo Mei (St) #5 (Daigei) is the connecting space of lower Yo Mei (St) myaku and upper Yo Mei (LI) myaku. Lower Yo Mei (St) #7 (Gekan) is the connecting space of lower Yo Mei (St) myaku and lower Sho Yo (GB) myaku. Upper Yo Mei (LI) #19 (Karyo) and upper Yo Mei (LI) #20 (Geiko) are also beneficial for teeth, gums, sinuses, and nerve issues. In addition, the thumb under the jaw stimulates the lymph nodes.

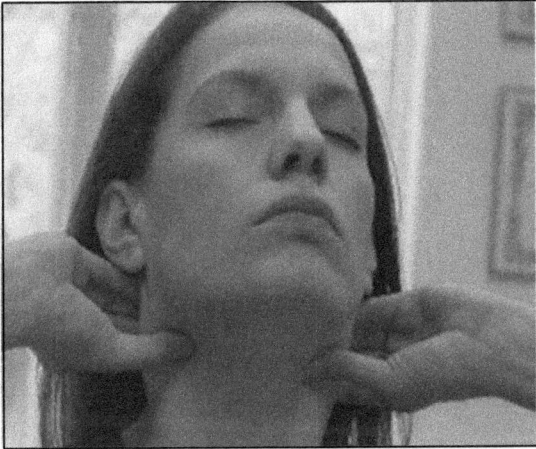

3) Nose and Face

Next, run your hands across the forehead from the center (medial) to the sides (lateral). Rub your eyebrows from medial to lateral. Rub the cheekbones with your thumb. Rub from the eye to the nose and outward under the maxillary bone. When massaging, follow along the contour of the bones. Rub under the nose and follow the maxillary bone from upper Yo Mei (LI) #20 (Geiko) to upper Sho Yo (TH) #17 (Eifu). There may be contractions on the upper Yo Mei myaku, under the cheekbone, if there are gum or teeth problems. From the ear, upper Sho Yo (TH) #17 (Eifu), press your thumb under and into the cheekbone and rub toward the mouth. Using four fingers, gently pull the skin of your face downward.

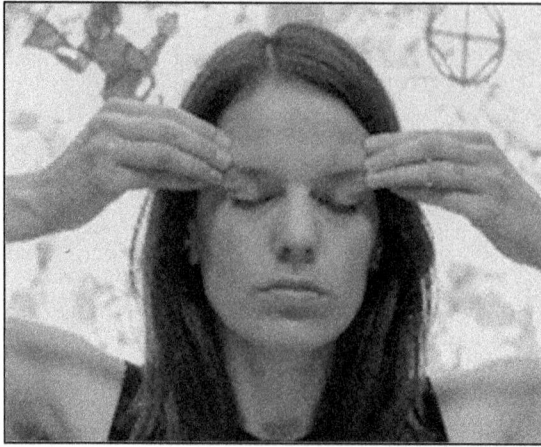

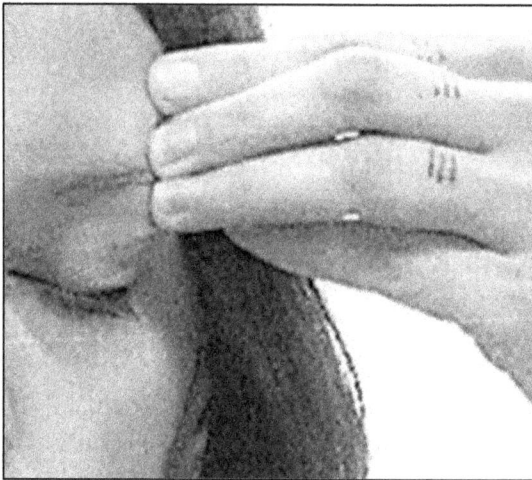

4) Eyes

Rub across the eyebrows in an outward direction, from Indo/Tokumyaku to lower Tai Yo (Bl) #2 *(Sanchiku)* to lower Sho Yo (GB) #14 *(Yohaku)*, upper Sho Yo (TH) #15 *(Tenryo)* and lower Sho Yo (GB) #1 (Doshiryo).

Rub softly around the eyes in an outward direction. Rub below the eyes in an outward direction.

Press the eyes directly with three fingers. Press on the eyelids until you "see lights," hold for a count of ten and release quickly, opening your eyes. Execute five times, opening your eyes each time you let go - helpful for eyesight, tension, and headaches. After pressing, rub your closed eyelids very softly, addressing nearsightedness and weak eyes; it tonifies the optical nerves and blood vessels. **5)** **Ears**

Pull your ears, stretching up from the top and down from the lobe, and bend the ears backward and forward. All myaku reach the ear; this is the basis of auricular therapy. Palpate the ear to find sensitive points and press where there is sensitivity. Rub hands over ears to increase circulation. Rub the skull below, on top, and behind the ears. Place a finger in the hole of both ear openings, vibrate your inserted finger, and pull out quickly. Do this several times: tonifies the ears, aids hearing issues and all other ear problems, unless you do it overenthusiastically and injure yourself.

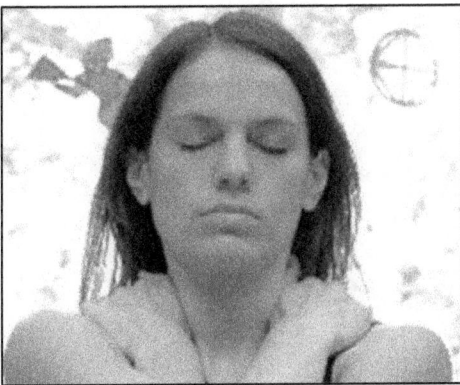

6)   Neck

Using four fingers, place next to the upper trapezius muscle and tendon at the back of the neck, next to the spine, press, and rock your head side to side. This area is the unique lower Tai Yo (Bl) #10 (Tenchu). Next, move fingers along the skull's base to lower the Sho Yo (GB) #20 (Fuchi) area. This movement affects the posterior vertebral muscles and the great auricular nerve. Repeat pressure and sideways rocking motion two to three times. Next, move out to lower Sho Yo (GB) #12 (Kankotsu) on the sternocleidomastoid muscle and repeat. Press with your thumb at the center of the junction of the spine and skull at Tokumyaku (GV) #15 (Amon). Rub along the top of the shoulders and neck. Lower Sho Yo (GB) #21 (Kankotsu) at the apex of the shoulder is a significant point suitable for high blood pressure, migraine, or cerebral vascular accident (CVA/stroke). For CVA, one <u>must</u> do handwork in this area. Strength is not needed. Do not use too much force; touching alone will have a pronounced effect. Never make the muscle "flip" or roll - too violent, not therapeutic. Place fingers on the side of muscles, not on top. The function is to remove contractions. Take your time. Be gentle; do not be greedy.

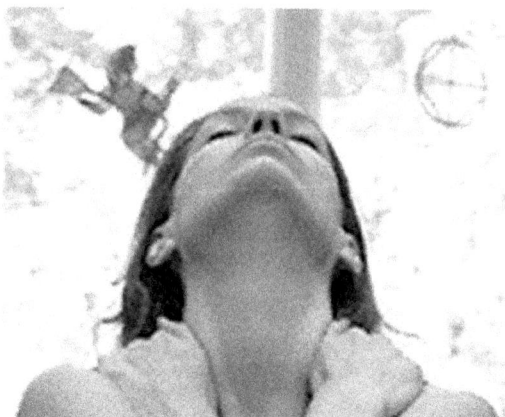

7)   Sides of neck

Place four fingers behind the sternocleidomastoid muscle, in line with upper Sho Yo (TH) #16 (Tenryo), and nod head front and back. Next, place your thumb in front of the muscle, in line with upper Tai Yo (SI) #17 (Tenyo), and rock your head back and forth. Do neck rolls and turns; always do exercises in both directions, clockwise and counterclockwise.

Rotate slowly, deeply yet gently, not quickly. This helps circulation to the brain and invigorates the cervical spine. Useful for tension, headaches, tonsillitis, swollen glands, and lymphatic stimulation.

8) Shoulders

In addition to addressing issues concerning the shoulders, these exercises help circulation to the head, arms, and hands and address issues involving the upper chest.

Because of internal organ conditions, shoulder muscles may interfere with circulation in the capillaries, resulting in blood not flowing adequately; numbness, pain, itching, and paralysis may occur. Blood not properly circulating to the head may manifest as high blood pressure, low blood pressure, headaches, migraines, ear problems, sinus problems, and eye issues. Blood not circulating down the arms may contribute to arthritis, rheumatism, skin problems, and numbness. This situation can also affect the nervous system; if blood circulation is inadequate, the nervous system might be compromised. Numbness and pain may come from a deficiency of the meridians.

Fever occurs when there is insufficient pressure to transport blood through the capillaries. Address the elasticity of the blood vessels; be assured of their tone. Blood flows from

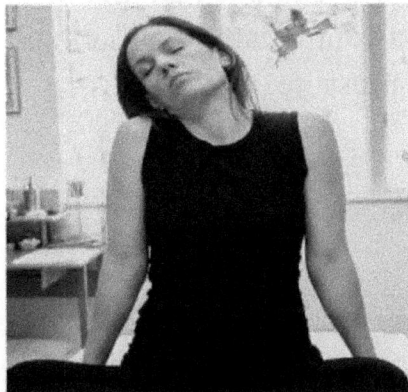

larger to smaller vessels; capillaries must pass the same amount as the aorta. If there are circulation problems, there can be blood pressure problems. Cerebral vascular issues may result.

Numbness and pain may come from a lack of flow in the shoulder. For relief and warming, rub along the meridians and bones.

a) Draw your shoulders up into your neck, relax, and let your shoulders drop; repeat at least five times.

b) Extend your head, cross your arms, and grasp the trapezius muscle at the shoulders, inhale and hold your breath, massage around the lower Sho Yo (GB) #21 (Kensei) area, exhale, and relax; repeat several times.

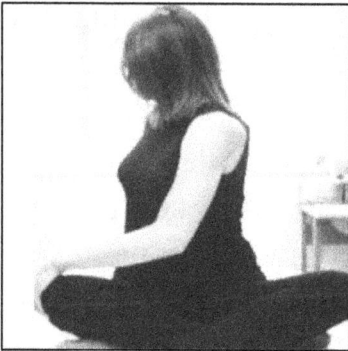

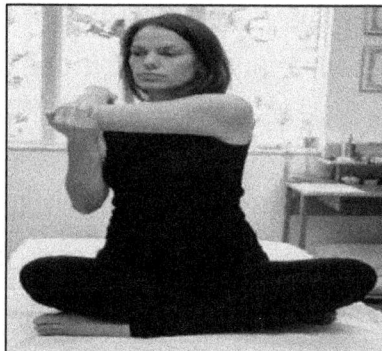

Fully extend the arms parallel to the earth; rotate your arms in both directions (clockwise and counterclockwise). This is essential to loosen the shoulders. Do this with a regular breathing pattern; do not hold your breath. Rotate arms in large loops and small loops. Draw shoulders up, head back, and move head side to side, ear to shoulder. Do this with a regular breath pattern; do not hold your breath. It aids circulation in the head and benefits blood pressure.

c) Rotate shoulders front to back, then reverse. While rotating your shoulders, roll your head in all directions. These are

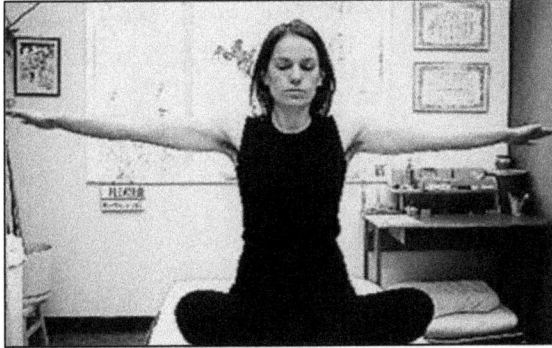

helpful for circulation in arms, hands, and joints.

d) While inhaling, extend the chest forward and draw the shoulders back; exhaling, let the chest and shoulders relax. Next, stretch the thoracic back and shoulders forward on inhale; exhale, let back, and relax shoulders. Repeat several times.

Push-ups are powerful for strengthening the shoulders and upper back. However, it is noteworthy that push-ups may be too muscular or too strong of a workout for many patients.

9) Arm

Cradle your elbow in the palm of your hand and pull the shoulder toward the center of the chest, rotating the upper body. If you are standing, align your feet to your ears.

Do each shoulder separately. Exhale at the end of the rotation; twist the upper spine, which is helpful for the upper spine and gives "shock" to the shoulder. Depending on your condition, do this while standing or sitting on the bed, chair, or floor. If you experience relief, rub along the bones to

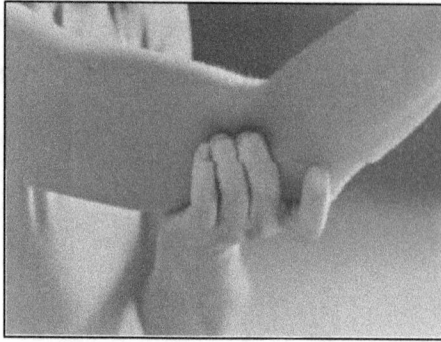

warm the meridians.

10) Elbow

Hold the triceps and brachioradialis muscles and swing the arm side-to-side. While holding the elbow, rotate, swing, and shake your hand. Then squeeze the forearm muscles while guiding the energy downward from the elbow to the wrist.

11) Wrist

Rub, squeeze, extend, flex, and bend your wrists in all contortions and directions.

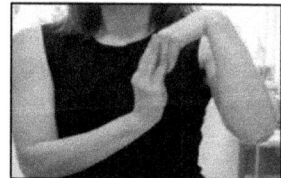

12) Hand

Massage each finger and rotate the joints; pulling the fingers is helpful for joint pain. Press down on the fingernails and the sides of the nails of each finger, this addresses tiredness. When you feel tired, squeeze your hand firmly.

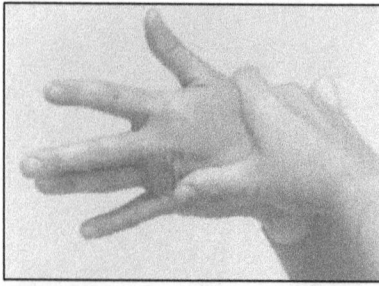
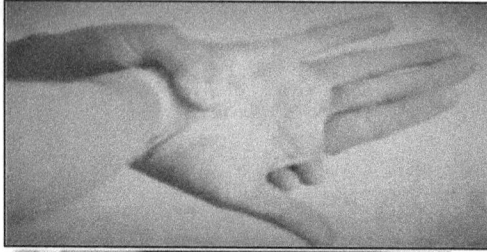
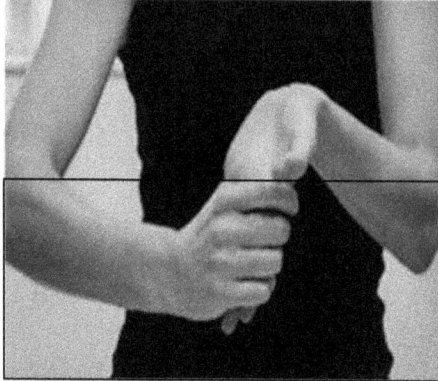
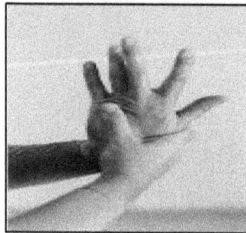

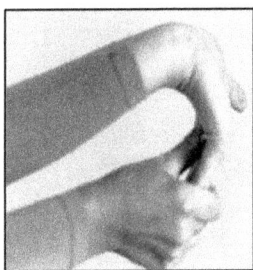
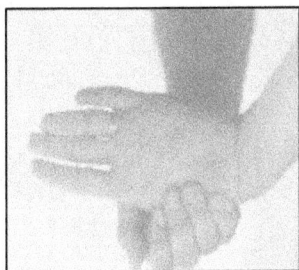
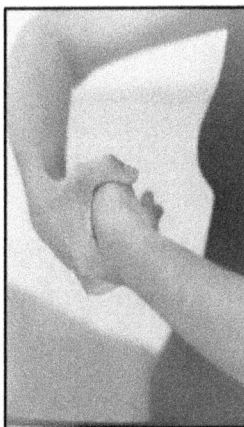
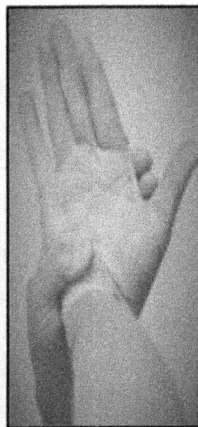
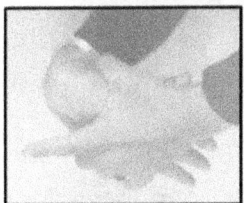
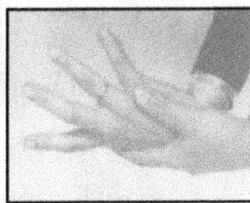
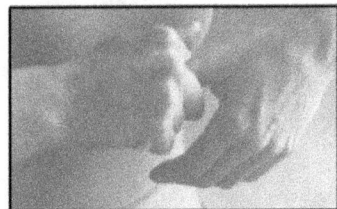
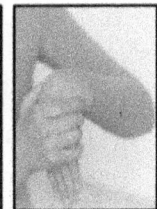

Use nail pressure on sei points. If overly sensitive, this indicates imbalances of that meridian. Press and massage the palm with your thumb. Press and squeeze your hands.

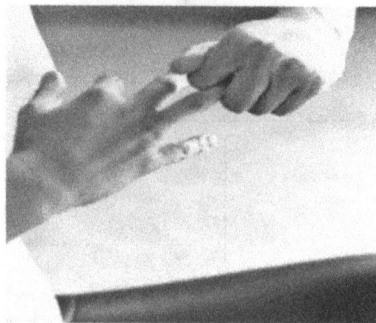

13) Torso

Chest: Energetically, we can become very stuck in the chest region. This area suffers from muscular tension in the back and neck. It holds the memory of lung contractions and congestion, muscular tension and trauma, emotional stresses, a "broken heart," and self-esteem issues.

The Bo/pooling point of the upper Tai Yin (Lu) #2 (Unmon) is an essential tsubo on the chest; it can be affected through upper Tai Yin (Lu) #6 (Kosai).

The Bo point of upper Ketsu Yin, Ninmyaku (CV) #17 (Danchu) can be affected at upper Ketsu Yin (HC) #3 (Kyokutaku).

These points are essential and can be immensely helpful for many conditions. If injury or modesty limits access to the chest, use points in the abdomen.

With teate, start at the center of the chest and work out. Follow the contours of the ribs and the flow of the skin. Pull gently on the ribs from the sternum. Note hot or cold temperatures, muscular contractions, or discomfort.

Use your four fingers on both hands. Cup your hands and grab the ribs from underneath with your fingers; lean over as you exhale. Catch the inside of the rib cage as you come back up. Pull apart and work the borders of the ribs. This affects the liver, gall bladder, heart, stomach, pancreas, and spleen. Pay attention to the sensations. Where are they going? What are they doing?

Place your hands overlapping to form a V and place above the pubic bone in front of the bladder. Lean forward as you are exhaling. Work on the sexual organs, bladder, and intestines. Choose sensitive points, work bilaterally, lean, and press. This treatment is significant for female issues— menstrual irregularity, menstrual cramps, menopausal discomfort, heavy flow, scanty flow, missed menses - any female problem. This treatment is also suitable for constipation, cramps, gas, and general toning of the reproductive and digestive systems.

14) Sides

Sitting with hands lightly resting on your knees, twist your torso and try to stick your head under your armpit, keeping your buttocks flat on the floor. Do this movement as you exhale; do a firm twist. Next, bend and rotate the torso from the hips.

Standing:

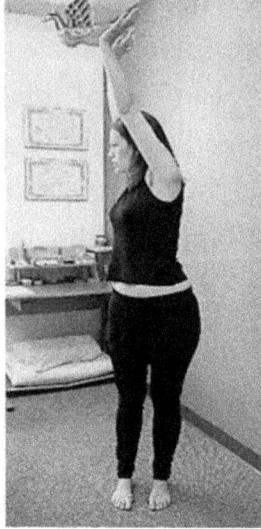

a) Sway your torso and head, side to side.
b) Place your hands on your hips, rotate the torso.

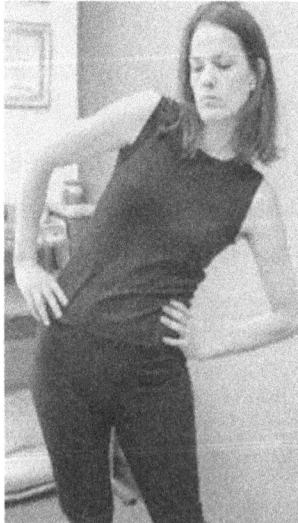

c) Raise your arms overhead; shake your hands and wrist, loose but not floppy Then with your palms upward, push the sky and rotate your torso. Always work bilaterally.

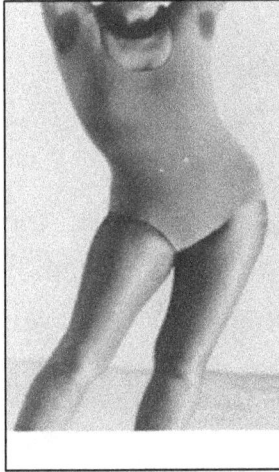

d) Push your fists into the lumbar region [lower Sho Yin (Kd) Yu area], bend backward and to the sides, leaning into the fists. Stretch forward while rocking on your toes, then swing your hips side to side for the spine.

e) Fists into hips and bend side to side.

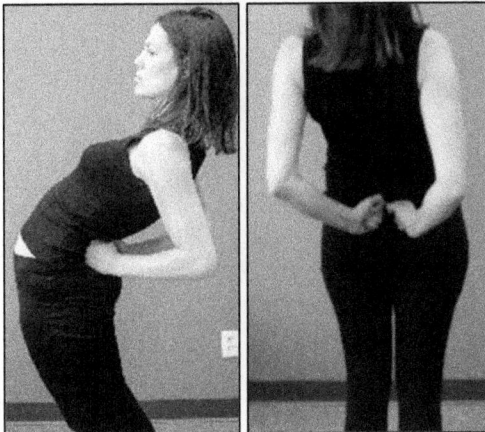

15) Hips

Deep knee bends (hold onto the wall if necessary).

Bend your knees, grab your knees, and rotate your hip, holding your knees.

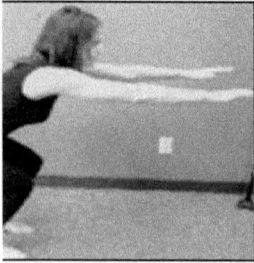

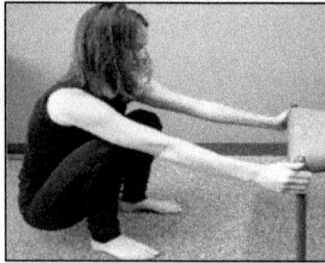

Stand on the balls of your feet and bounce on your toes with your knees flexed (deep knee bend position). This benefits the hips, lower back, legs, knees, and circulation. Muscle tension in the thighs is related to the

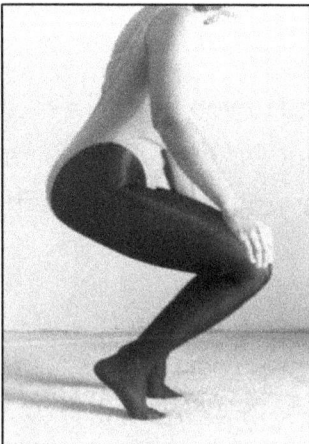

stomach. When addressing digestive issues, we must do teate to the hips
and thighs.

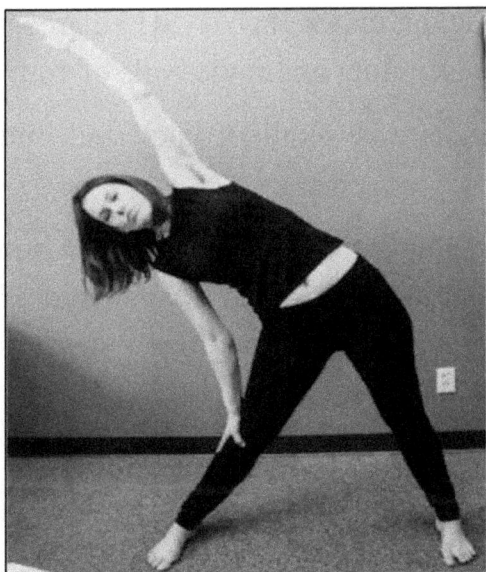

Standing, spread one leg laterally, raise the opposite arm overhead, both feet flat. Stretch by sliding your hand down the outstretched leg, first with the other foot flat, and then allow the foot on the side with the outstretched arm to "roll" to the outside and hyper-extend, not too hard.

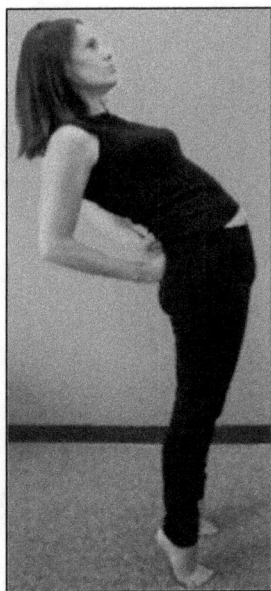

Standing, fists in the sacral region, upper Tai Yo (SI) Yu area, bend back, and stretch your legs by standing up on the balls of your feet.

Standing, pound fists on thighs and small of back and buttock, helpful for circulation.

Diamond Exercise: Sitting on your bottom, sitting with the bottom of your feet touching each other in front, forming a diamond. Place your hands on the top of your feet, cupping your toes, pull the heels toward your crotch, elbows pressing on your knee.

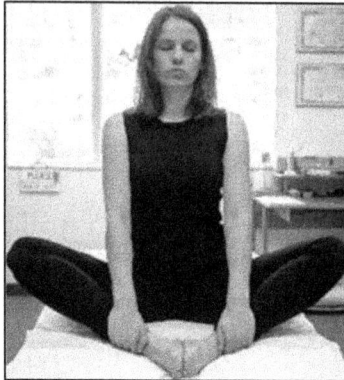

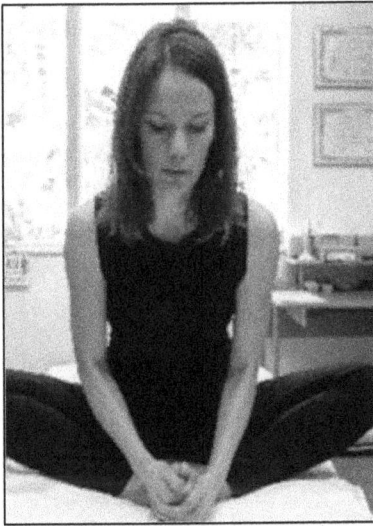

Bounce knees up and down. This act stretches the inside of the thighs and is good for hip joints. Stiff or tight hip joints can be the cause of many problems. You must keep the hips flexible. This exercise also opens the junction of the hip and groin, where the femoral artery is located, helping circulation to the lower extremities.

16) Legs, Knees, Feet

Sitting with your legs straight, keep heels in place and flex feet toward each other, big

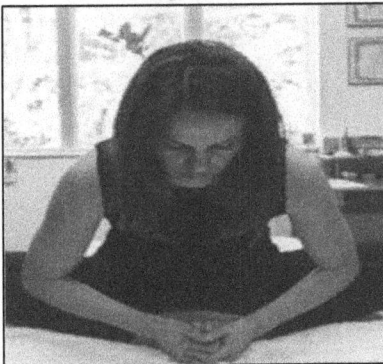

toes touching. Relax your feet. Reach toward the ankle, one leg at a time,

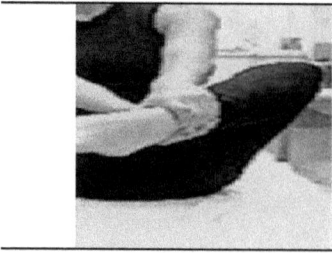

and stretch the torso down the leg. Grab your ankle if you

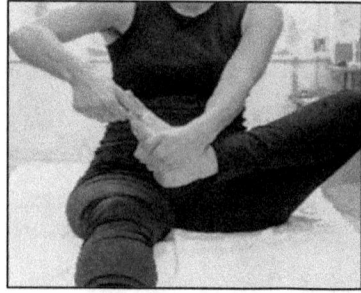

can. If not, extend as far as possible. Repeat the exercise with your other
leg.

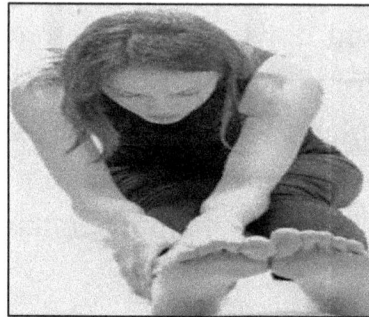

In the same position as above, grab your leg below the knee and rotate the leg and ankle. Hold your ankle at lower Sho Yin (Kd) #3 (Taikei) and turn the ankle clockwise and counterclockwise. Massage your foot and toes; pull your toes. Hold your ankle and shake your foot.

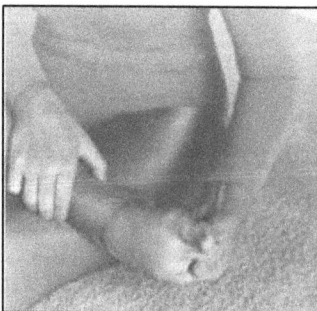

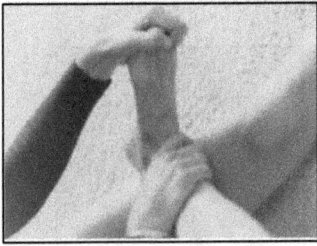

Work the feet; hold, rub, pinch each toe, and massage sensitive and sei points. Use nail pressure on the sei points. The sensitivity indicates imbalances of that meridian. Next, press the sole with your thumb, like teate to the palm. Repeat on the other leg and foot.

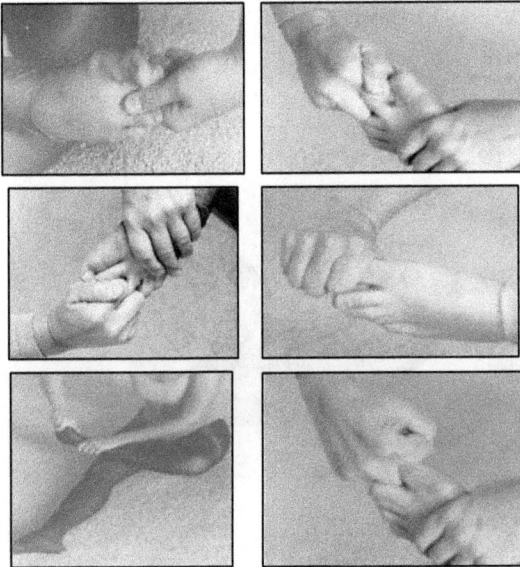

17) Lower Back and Abdomen

Lying on your back,

> a. Hip Roll (for digestion and circulation): RELAX. Flex knees with feet on the floor and roll hips from side to side using the weight of the knees. Keep your back flat

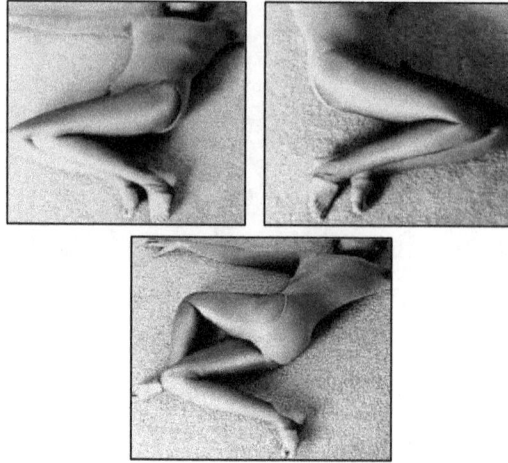

B With your feet flat on the floor, lift your hips, arch your back, and kick your legs up and out, landing solidly on your sacral spine - helps the hips and kidneys.

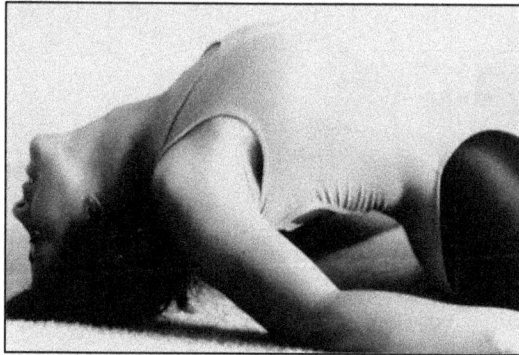

b. To tone your abdomen, lie on your back with your legs straight. Clasp your hands behind your head. Drop your elbows to the floor. Raise your right knee out to the side and bring it up to touch your right elbow. All movements occur on the exhale. Hold for one breath cycle. Return to lying flat. Now the left leg. Repeat ten times on each side. Keep your body flat on the floor - tonifies the lateral aspect of your torso and elongates the sacrum and lumbar spine.

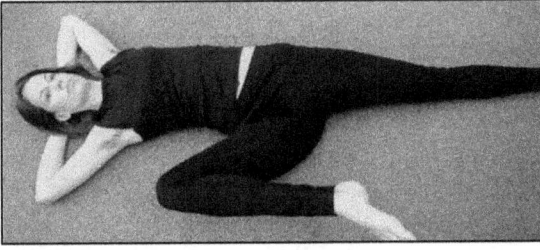

Cobra Exercise: Lie on your stomach, with your hands at your side, or place your hands to form a triangle in front of your face: Raise your head, shoulders, and upper back with your back muscles; do not push with your arms—this tonifies from lower Sho Yo Bo to upper Yo Mei Yu tsubo and the

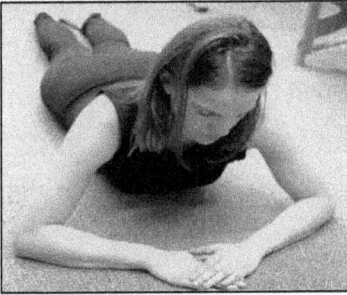

abdomen.

19) Upper Back and Neck

Head-Shoulder Curl: Lie on your back with your knees bent. Clasp your hands behind your neck and gradually raise your head off the floor. Next, raise your shoulders until they are about ten inches off the floor. Then, slowly lower yourself back down. Repeat ten times, rest one minute, and repeat ten more times.

"The Golden Fish": Lie on your back, head up with hands clasped behind your head— wiggle on your back, with a wavy, spiral motion, like a fish. Move in the direction of your head; do not stay in one place.

The Final Touch:

Lie on your stomach and kick your buttocks with the heels of your feet; this aids the abdomen and thighs; because it loosens thigh muscles, it relaxes the core.

Lie on your back with your feet flat, knees flexed, and hips up. Bounce from your feet and thoracic back. You are vibrating the internal organs.

RELAX

These exercises are for self-healing. Work on yourself always. It would be best if you mastered these exercises before showing anyone else how to use them. It would be best if you guided each patient based on your self-experience. Remove contractions, work on meridians, nerves, blood and lymph circulation, muscles, joints, intestines, sexual organs, digestive organs—all organs. Work on feeling good, relaxation, happiness, and wholeness.

By beginning with yourself, you can learn to guide others through your experience, focusing on the points, contractions, sensations, and responses of self. With selfwork, just as when treating another, ONE MUST GO SLOW. Hand Qi perceives energy. With the greater practice of hand Qi, comes greater perception. Hand Qi may awaken self-will while synchronizing energetically to all body parts, which happens accidentally or purposefully. Know what you are doing.

It would be best if you took sickness out slowly. One's own Life Energy, IE dimension (life-will empowered), is the healer. Feel what you are doing with self-work, just as with work on the patient. Identify trouble spots. If some part of the meridian, nervous, or circulatory system is off, it will manifest somewhere on the meridians. LOOK FOR IT!!! Find the stagnation and alter it.

Where is it? What is it? Cold skin is the cause or symptom of many kinds of imbalance. Try to make all mistakes in diagnosis and treatment on yourself. To work on others, one must always be working on self.

CHAPTER NINE

TEATE TREATMENT

WITH MOXIBUSTION AND HARI

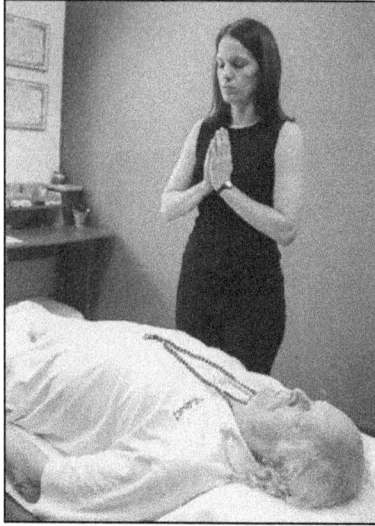

Work on "other" from your tanden. Keep your knees relaxed, unlocked, neither bent nor flexed. Maintain your energy flow from your center of gravity, your tanden. Stay grounded. Operate from your tanden. Always start with hand Qi exercise. Touch your partner the same way you touch your hands when practicing hand Qi exercises. Handwork allows the patient to heal themselves; the practitioner is assisting in recovering and maintaining the balance of their energy.

TEATE TREATMENT

Circulation is vital. Stagnation in small vessels causes rashes, varicose veins, shingles, staph infections, headaches, fuzzy thinking, and the like. Office workers need energetic work on the head, neck, shoulders, and upper back; physical workers tend to lose their energy through the lower back, hips, and abdomen. Consider how the patient uses their body when planning treatment.

When treating a patient, seek to assist that person in achieving an 80 percent balance; the patient must do at least 20 percent of the work. Do not seek a 100 percent balance. That will exhaust the patient and cause that person to depend on you for stability. What nonsense! Who wants such a control freak for a physician? Allow the patient to focus on the point, contractions, and sensations. Handwork does not cure. The hand awakens the patient's self-will while conveying energy to the parts of the body. One's own Life-Energy (I dimension) is the healer. We are just helping. Go slow. Be a servant.

Have patient work on self, but do not force it! How much? Each patient is different. You must judge how much, and what dosage. Do not try to remove multi-contractions at once.

Abdomen

Begin perpendicular to your partner. Always begin with a gentle laying of the palm on tanden. Next, remind your partner to breathe into the lower abdomen. When working on the abdomen, start in the center, work from the inner to the outer (medial to lateral), and return to the center.

141

Sakai Sensei treated all conditions in the abdomen; any illness of mind-body-spirit, he remedied within the hara.

Ampuku (Calm the Abdomen) Abdominal Rubbing Strokes

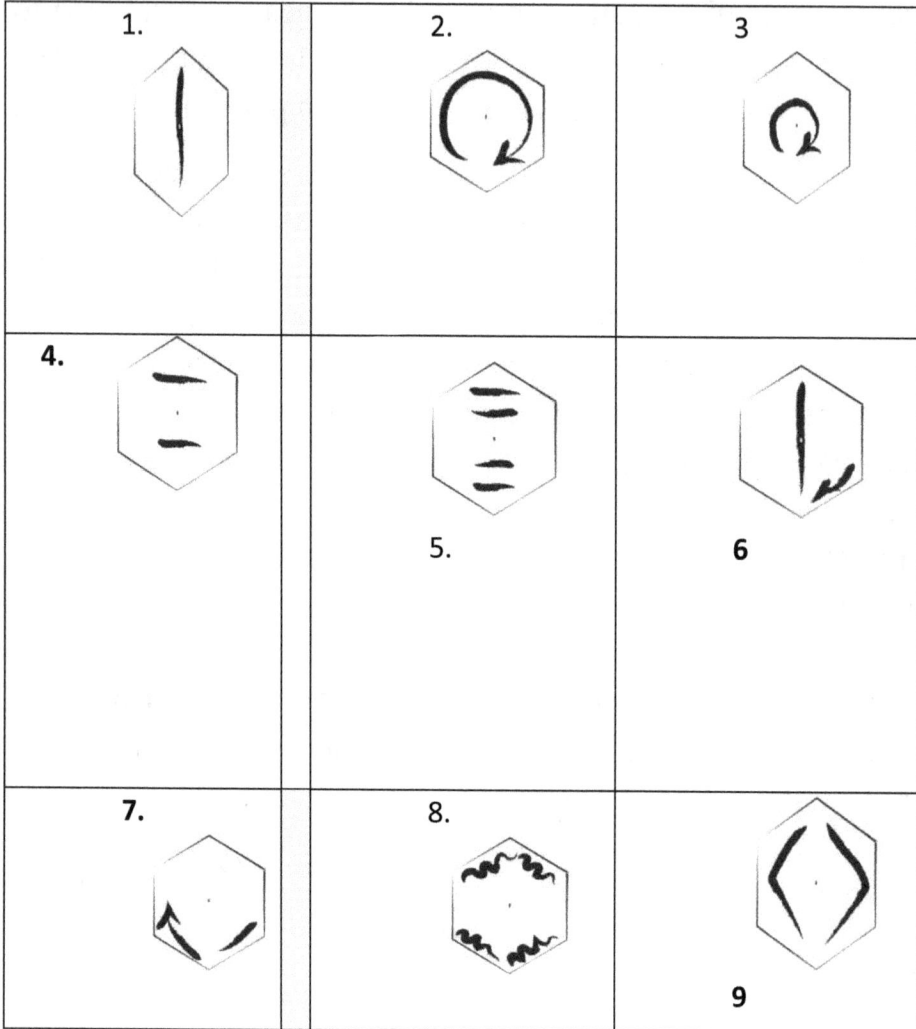

1.	2.	3
4.	5.	6
7.	8.	9

Based on diagnosis:

1. Heart/Shimpo/ Jo Sho
2. Large Intestine
3. Spleen/Stomach

4. Blood, Large Intestine/Small Intestine
5. Blood/digestion/Large Intestine/Small Intestine
6. Shimpo/Kidney/Gall Bladder
7. Gall Bladder/Intestine
8. Liver/Heart/Spleen/Small Intestine/Bladder/Large Intestine
9. 9 Diamond: Whole System:
   Inguinal/Costal/Heart/Heart
   Constrictor/Kidney/Bladder/Small
   Intestine/Large Intestine/Liver/Gall Bladder

Abdominal Teate

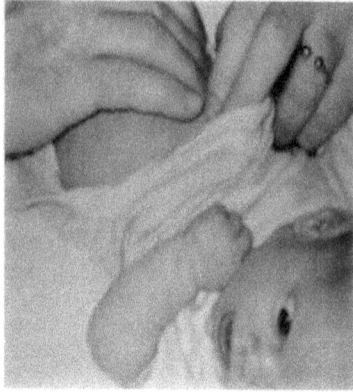

Younger

Older

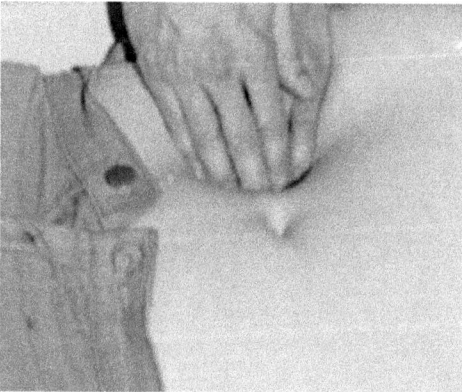

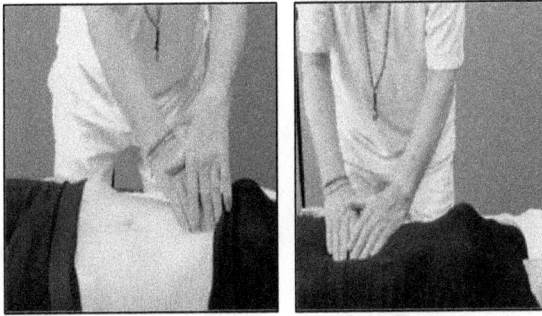

Start below the tip of the xiphoid process at Ninmyaku (CV) #15 (Kyubi) with the fingertips of one hand on top of the fingers of the other. Work your way down the center abdominal line to the navel, Ninmyaku (CV) #8 (Shinketsu), then down from the navel to the edge of the pubic bone, Ninmyaku (CV) #2 (Kyokotsu). Keep your fingers aligned and your hands parallel. Do not press the navel directly; it is not comfortable.

Reach across the abdomen. Cup your fingers and place them on the side of the abdomen between the iliac crest and below the ribs. Then, with a cupping motion, press inward toward the center abdominal line, Ninmyaku (CV).

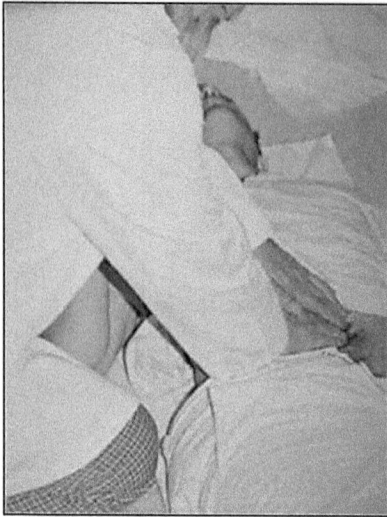

Osensei illuminating Sakai Teate

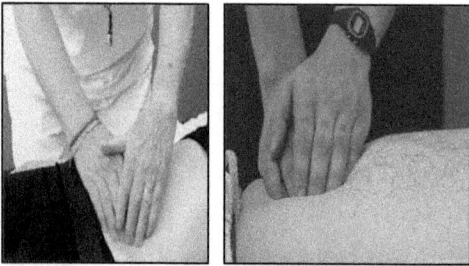

Gather data here; note everything through your fingertips and visual observation. Brush away ju, floating stagnation that is accumulating.

Note deep stagnation (shaku); note body temperature, moisture, and pain sites.

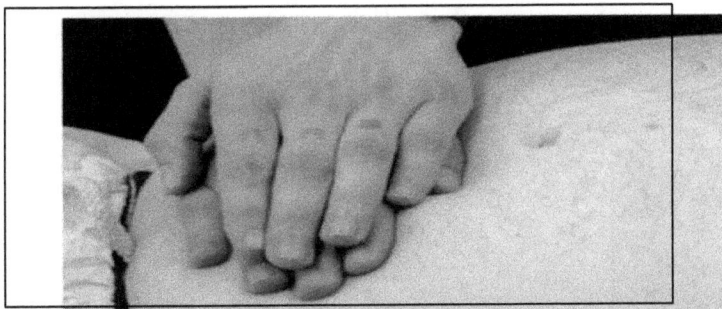

Working on the side of the person's abdomen furthest from you, cup your fingers to pull the physical and energetic abdomen toward the center. Working on the side of the person's abdomen closest to you, use your thumbs for cupping and push in toward the center.

Work toward the center on the front, even when moving away from the center. Work out from the center on the back.

Using fingertips on top of fingers, reach across, starting on the opposite side of the person's abdomen. Begin at the top of the wing of the ilium and move upward, following the curve of the patient's abdomen towards the ribs to the xiphoid process. Then, come back down to the wing of the ilium on the near side, down the inguinal area to the pubis, across the edge of the pubic bone, and back to the ilium where you began—a full circle with your hands following the contour of the arch of the ribs and pelvic bone. Provide specific abdominal teate to address the issues encountered. When sinking deeper into the abdomen, let your fingers travel as the patient exhales. When you locate contractions, exert pressure on the exhale, release on the inhale, from your tanden, not physical strength! This is a sha-type gesture. Hold your position while the patient is inhaling. Do not retreat; hold that position. When you are ready to move away from that spot, do so on the patient's exhalation.

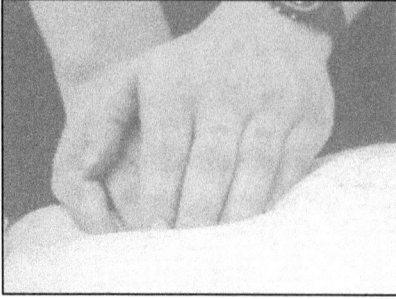

When working the line below the navel, ask the patient to remove or undo buckles and buttons. Do not press on top of objects that may cause discomfort or alter your pressure.

Back

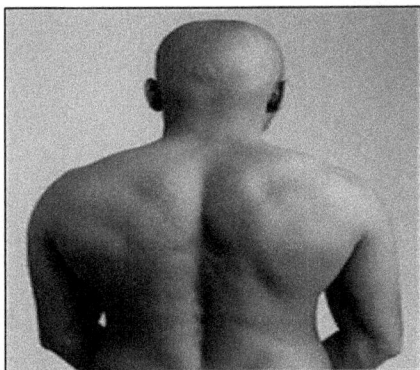

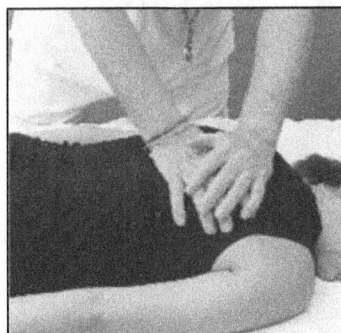

Elimination of Ju: Next, with the patient in the prone position, stimulate Qi to flow on the back with light shiatsu-style teate for several minutes. When you feel the Qi flowing, palpate the back-yu points and third line and provide kyu on tender points until reddening appears. [If performing hari, provide light tapping on the skin without twirling the needle for a minute or so until the ju is gone. There is no need to pierce the surface, but if that happens, it is okay.] Continue with light tapping until faint redness appears. Reddening may not occur.

Pay attention; do not overtreat.

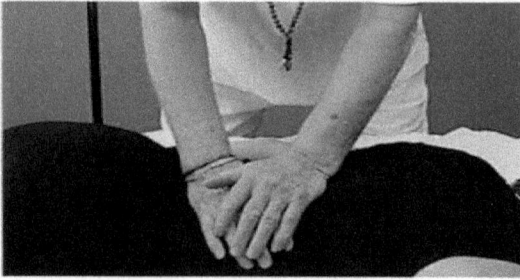

Elimination of Shaku: Based on abdominal shaku diagnosis, use teate and needling for five seconds on all tender points on the back in the corresponding areas of shaku findings. [Needling is very shallow and provided on the first, second, and third bladder lines and Tokumyaku. Needling is from medial to lateral.]

When the back treatment is complete, recheck the abdomen for the shaku you have been addressing to determine the efficacy of the treatment. You may apply teate or needling until you experience the arrival of hibiki.

Back Teate
Place one hand flat on the other and push down the spine from the top of the thoracic spine to the bottom of the sacral spine in small sweeping motions. Make a tactile and visual observation of the shape, configuration, and alignment of the vertebrae

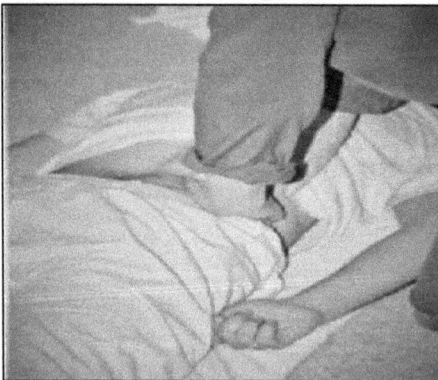

to each other and the center of the spine.

Reach across your patient's back, place the pad of your thumb in the groove along the side of the spinal column, and press that thumb with the heel of your other hand. Run your thumb down the side of the spine, in the vertebral groove, from top to bottom, with firm pressure on the side of the spine, providing a quick sweeping motion. Drain that groove of blockages. Go down one side of the spine, next to the vertebrae, and then treat the other side. This is considered the first bladder line; a half tsun from the spine in their respective locations are the pediatric yu points. All the points five bu on either side of the vertebrae may be treated with shonishin, needles, or moxa.

Now work down the left and right sides of the back, one and a half tsun from the spine, two fingers width, the classic bladder line, and yu points; then repeat the therapy down the back, about four fingers, three tsun, distance from the spine. When treating back yu points, include the third line if the condition is chronic; the site shows shaku, or the tsubo depicts an "alert" state. When attending the yu points, pay attention to correspondences. The upper zo yu points on the upper back correspond to the upper fu yu points on the lower back. The communications of zo yu points on the posterior to zo bo points on the anterior torso. Upper and lower, front and back, inline and diagonal—allow the relationships to guide you. All locations are vital.

Tokumyaku (GV) #12 (Shinchu): Treat children with moxa for all issues above the diaphragm.

Tokumyaku (GV) #4 (Meimon):
    For all diseases below the diaphragm.

Tokumyaku (GV) #3 (Koshi no Yokan): For issues relating to the harmony of Tokumyaku (GV)/Ninmyaku (CV)

Tokumyaku (GV) #2 (Yoyu): Bladder discord may result in renal or cardiac insufficiency.

The Abnormal Spine: In cases where the condition is more functional than organic, the muscles in the gutter of the spine will tend to be tense and constricted, and the external tissues will be soft. With organic disease, the trough of the spine and the superficial muscles will be ropey, constricted, tender, and painful. Where the organ or organs are atonic, lacking strength or power, the gutter of the spine will be soft and puttylike, and the external muscles will be ropey.

I treated my first multiple sclerosis patient with the guidance of Nakazono Osensei. He instructed me to push the "putty " toward the coccyx through repetitious sessions. Then, based on pulse diagnosis, I treated her twice a week, providing hari, kyu, kappo, and teate, with attention to the spinal region, as Osensei instructed. This patient went from wheelchair to walker to cane to unassisted walking to dance school to opening a school— an unusual case. With my multiple sclerosis patients, I have paid much attention to this kind of spinal care and balancing the pulses. I have had incredibly positive results with some and no adverse effects with any. People with scoliosis also benefit from considerate teate to the spinal section of the body and abdominal teate.

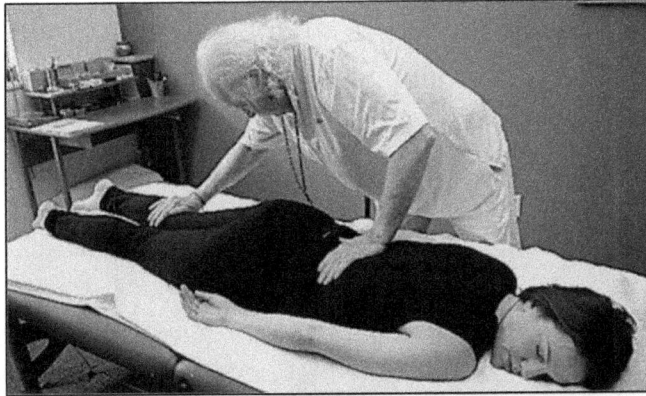

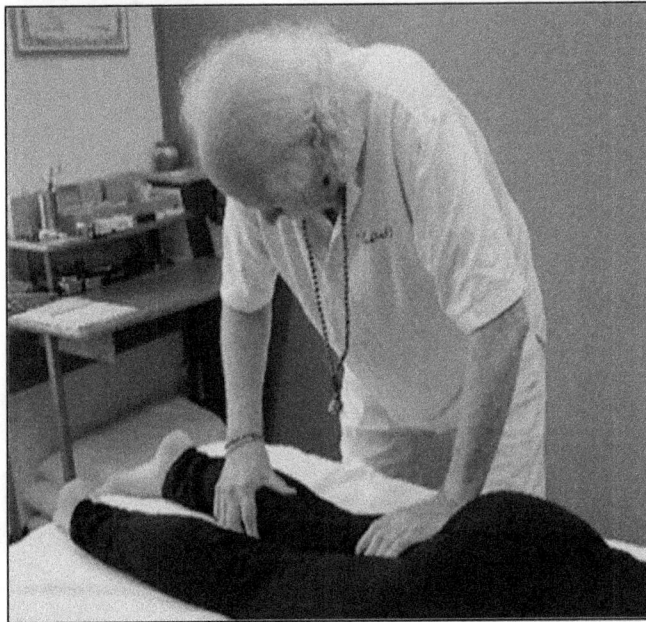

<u>Hamstrings</u>: While the patient is prone, ensure the patient's legs align relative to the spine. Do this by pointing the large toe of each foot toward the other. With the feet flat, the balls of the feet turned upward, and the toes turned inward, the spine naturally self-aligns. Standing, place one foot directly below the buttock on the lower gluteus maximus muscle, the arch of your foot caressing the crease of the buttock and thigh. Place the

other foot in the same position on the other leg. Maintain your center and balance in tanden. From tanden, use a rocking motion from side to side, slowly shifting your weight from hip to hip while keeping the triangulation of your legs to your tanden. Allow your feet to lightly stimulate your patient's hip joints, muscles, and meridians.

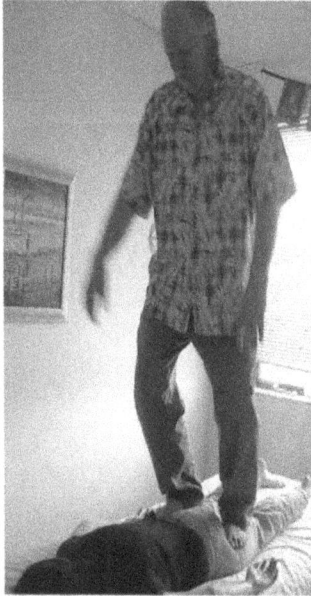

Before stepping off your patient's thigh, you may step up onto the buttock with the knees slightly bent and the large toes bilateral to the sides of L5. Standing thus, perform three deep knee bends from your tanden. If you cannot be in your tanden, do not attempt this. To come out of this position, aise one foot and step to your patient's side as you both are exhaling.

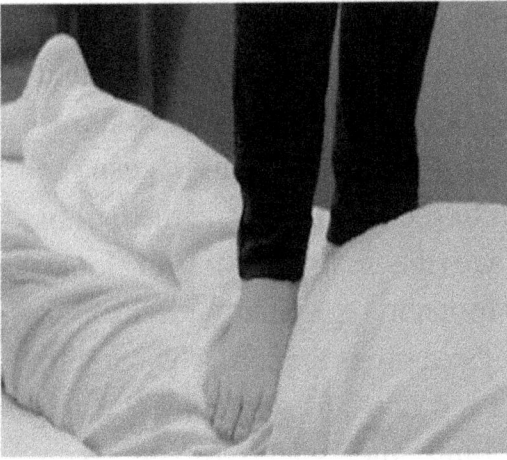

DO NOT STEP BACKWARD

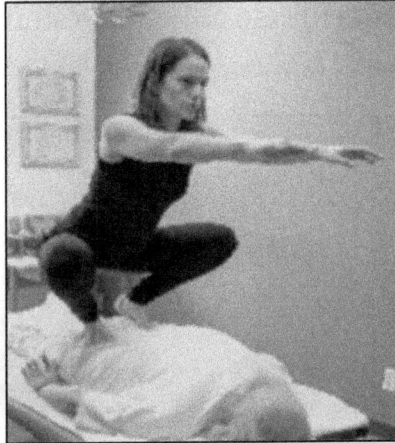

<u>Feet Walk:</u> Stand between the patient's legs facing outward. Place the arch of your right foot on the arch of your patient's right foot; distribute your weight through the balls of your feet. Place the arch of your left foot on the juncture of the patient's Achilles tendon and calcaneus. You are always facing outward.

Establish a gentle rocking motion with the hips from tanden through your legs, with your weight distributed through the balls of your feet. With that motion, allow your left foot to walk up that tendon and gently cusp the calf muscle with the arch of the left foot while the ball of the foot is on a solid surface (the treatment table or floor), providing support to the foot and leg). Start with the arch of your foot on the patient's Achilles tendon. Always start from below the patient's leg muscles and complete the movement before reaching the knee. Never exert pressure on the back of the knee.

To exert pressure evenly, distribute your pressure by stepping, more like rocking, from side to side rather than straight downward. You need, through your tanden, to distribute your weight

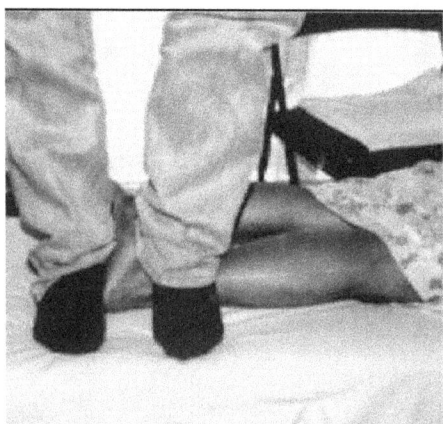

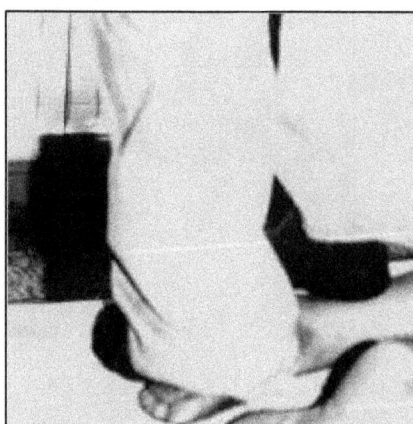

throughout your body to allow your patient to relax.

To disembark from this position, raise the foot contacting the Achilles tendon and step laterally to your patient's side as you both are exhaling.

DO NOT STEP BACKWARD!

While standing between your patient's legs, place your left foot on the back of your patient's right knee, reach down, take the patient's right foot, and bend the leg to a 90- degree angle, hold the foot with both hands, stabilize leg with the left foot and as the patient exhales, pull the foot upward to stretch ankle.

These maneuvers are stretching the tissue, enhancing the patency of the meridians', and expanding energy as it flows down the leg into the foot.

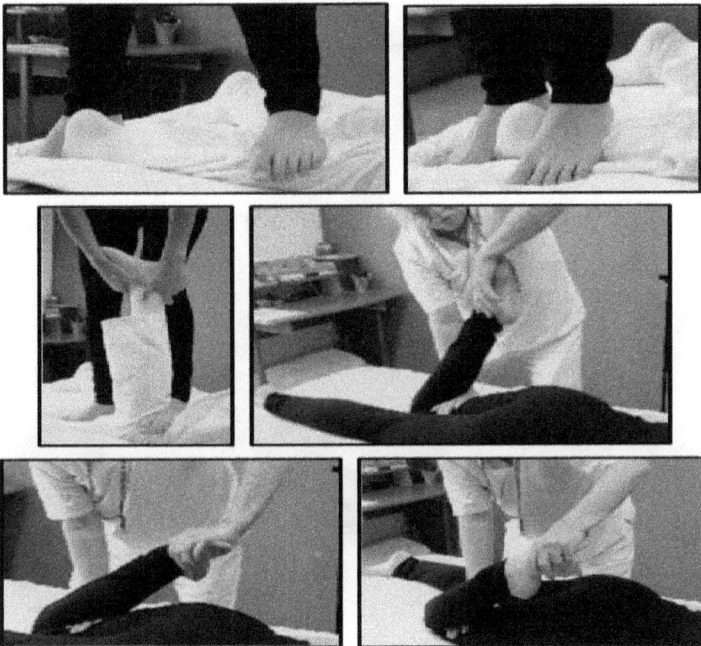

Hips and Side

This effect opens the lower Sho Yin myaku and awakens the lower Tai Yo and lower Tai Yin myaku. There is immediate access to lower Sho Yin, lower Tai Yo, lower Ketsu Yin, and lower Yo Mei. These meridians allow access to the entire nervous, digestive, reproductive, and circulatory systems, the Achilles tendon, and all tendons and ligaments in the front of the patient's foot.

The patient lies on the side, facing you. You want your patient to be comfortable and linear but natural.

Straighten your patient's legs with the knee slightly bent. Keep the patient's legs extended so as not to inhibit full stretch, place the arm that the patient is lying on under their head. Knees slightly bent are more natural but be careful; the bent knee may work as a wedge and interfere with the stretching motion.

Arrange the hip in this position first, then control the shoulder. Next, using cupping motion and the side of the hand, work the area of the iliac crest: around, above, back, top, and front of it, connecting with the lower Sho Yin yu points, upper Yo Mei yu points, and lower Sho Yo myaku.

Place the opposite arm behind the body. Your patient should not move their arm; this causes contraction of muscles. The patient is passive; the provider is active

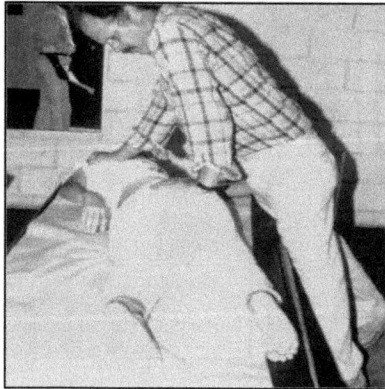

As pictured above, push your patient's hip inward in a spiral motion; push the shoulder outward in the opposite spiral motion while the patient exhales. You move in a spiral, turning from your tanden. Stretch following the natural line of the body. The movement asks the body to

open from its tanden. Implement on the opposite side as well.

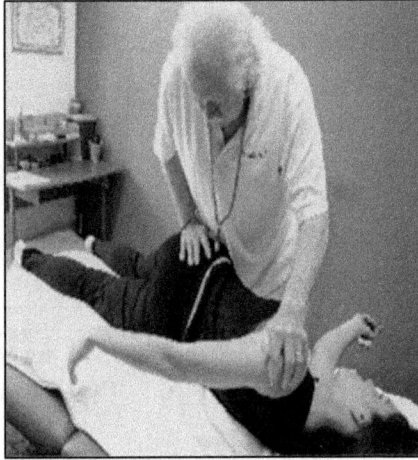

Back and Spine

Have your patient sit up. Kneel behind your patient. Adjust the height of your body to align your chest with your patient's back at the site you wish to stretch. You may have to adjust your leg sitting to raise or lower your body to achieve the correct alignment.

Maneuvering the back, take your patient's hands and place one on top of the other on the back of their head. Do not allow the patient to put their hands on their head; that creates muscular tension. The patient needs to be passive.

Reach under the patient's armpit, fold your arms back through the patient's arm, and clasp your hands on the top of your patient's clasped hands, one on top of each other.

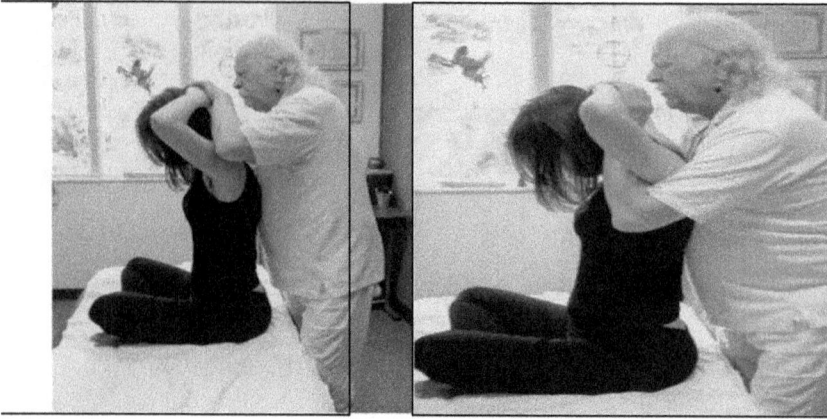

DO NOT LEAN FORWARD ONTO THE PATIENT.
DO NOT CAUSE THE PATIENT TO LEAN FORWARD.

Have the patient inhale and fill their chest with air; their back will become slightly concave. Inhale simultaneously, causing your chest to expand, filling in the open space as your patient inhales. Patient and practitioner function as one unit; the practitioner is inhaling and begins to arch back as the patient inhales. Instruct the patient to exhale.

Delay your exhalation by half a breath so that your chest will maintain contact with the patient's back. The practitioner exhales with the patient. The practitioner moves upward and arches back as the patient exhales; it is one arch, providing a full inline stretch. These are mechanical movements synchronized in breath and action, but the essence of our kappo is within tanden. It is not automatic; it is energetic. Coordinate all stretches and other maneuvers with the patient's breathing. The practitioner should quietly synchronize the breathing with the other person and move in coordination with the patient. When a patient inhales a yin action, and the practitioner causes the patient to expand, a yang action, by applying kappo, pressure, or body movement, that movement will be against the patient's life principle, and the patient will be hurt. Do not ask your patient to synchronize with you; that is backward. You should synch your breathing and your actions to your patient's.

Shoulder and Neck

Stand behind your patient with your thumbs pressing into the shoulders at lower Sho Yo (GB) #21 *(Kensei)*. You are asking the patient's shoulders to relax by lightly shocking them. Be aware of the cervical spine communicating with the head.

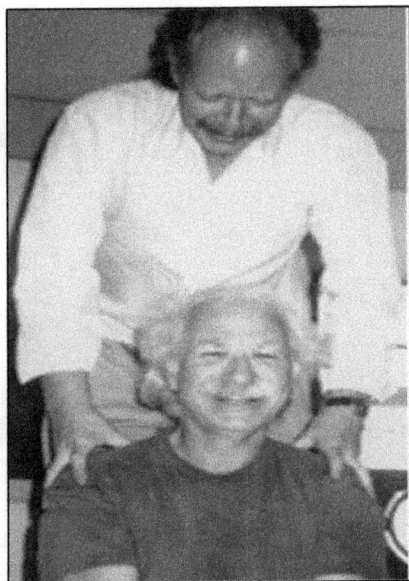

On the shoulders are lower Sho Yo (GB) tsubo, upper Yo Mei (LI) tsubo, upper Tai Yo (SI) tsubo, and upper Sho Yo (TH) tsubo. With hands and fingers, stimulate these points. In addition, rubbing the lateral aspect of the upper arms has proven an effective treatment procedure for reproductive organ issues.

Cervical Stretching: To stretch the cervical spine and musculature to the left and right, cup your left hand under the basilar aspect of the skull (occipital region at the lower back of the head); cup your right hand under the chin. Position your right knee to create contact between your knee and the right side of your patient's back. Use your hands to cradle the head and chin. With the arms turning the head—cupping, not grabbing, not shoving—provide mild torque. Observe your patient's breathing and synchronize your breathing with your patient's breathing pattern. On the exhale, pull the head up and twist to the right. The patient needs a pivotal point to turn. Use your leg and knee to provide that fixed position to pivot around. If turning to the right, use the right knee against the patient's right shoulder to maintain the patient's trunk and hip alignment with knee stability.

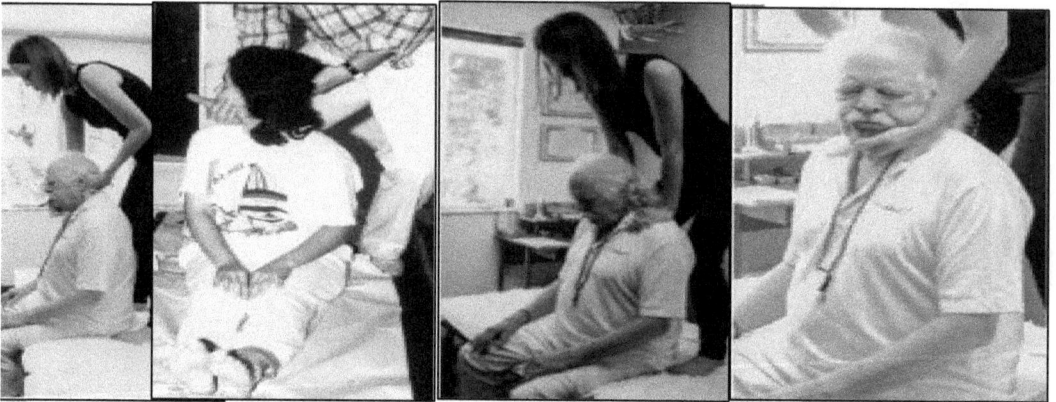

Change hands and repeat on the other side: right hand below the skull, left hand under the chin before turning left, left knee against the left shoulder as a stabilizer.

Finish with either the index or middle finger sliding from upper Yo Mei (LI) #20 (Geiko) along the cheekbone to upper Sho Yo (TH) #17 (Eifu). Then, slide along the top of the eye orbit with the same fingers; thumbs are above the eyebrow, applying pressure from the forehead to the temple. Push the center of the head down with the fingertips of both hands. Rub the head. Soft spots, a sign of water stagnation, are drained by teate. Remember, chronic conditions usually take a prolonged time to recover and repair.

KAPPO –
Giving Back Life First Aid, Revival, Resuscitation
"Take Back" Techniques

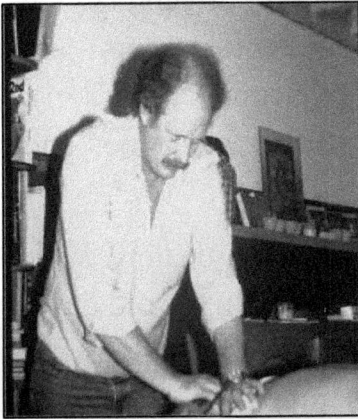

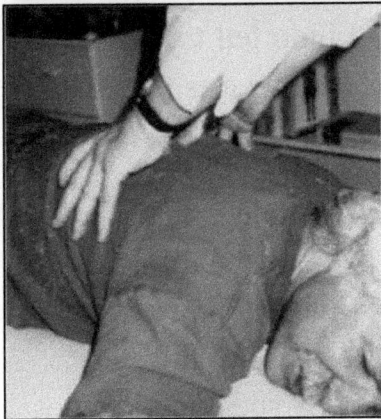

From the "barefoot doctors" of rural China to the paramedics throughout the world, from the Native traditional healer to the

Japanese martial arts kappo master, first aid and emergency care have been studied and applied in every setting throughout the world and throughout history.

From early history until now, all knowledge and skills in trauma care developed in warfare. From the development of the ambulance (Napoleonic Wars, 1802) to the traction splint (WWI) to burn trauma (WWII) and posttraumatic shock syndrome and toxic environmental poisons (Vietnam), our capacity to care for injuries has closely followed our ability to inflict injuries.

As with most systems of medicine, oriental medicine has various branches and specialties. As far back as the eighth century, the Japanese government established training requirements and licensing for some branches. These included acupuncture (hari), herbalism (kampo), pediatrics, surgery, internal medicine, and bodywork (teate).

One aspect of teate—kappo—was the specialty dealing with skeletal and muscular issues and soft tissue injury. In the old days, these specialists, "bonesetters," marketed their disciplines. In modern times, they would be osteopathic therapists.

Nakazono Osensei's training in kendo and judo led to his kappo studies in 1936, and that training led to the healing arts, especially acupuncture, diet, and teate.

Traditional medicine appreciates holism, the whole greater than its parts, and the interrelationships of the components. When encountering chronic trauma, there is much more going on than just a symptom. There is a need to know the cause of this symptom. If the causative factors, energetically speaking, are not addressed, the symptoms will return, worsen, or change to a more profound, more severe condition. With acute trauma, the extent of the injury must be determined so rapid and complete recovery can take place.

X-rays, blood tests, or other mechanical diagnostic devices may be beneficial. However, there is much more from the viewpoint of traditional medicine; there are injuries to Qi and blood, the underlying energetics of life.

Trauma usually creates bi syndrome or obstruction. This is because the injury usually involves excessive energy, which disturbs the flow of Qi and blood. When some excessive force causes capillaries or larger blood vessels to rupture, the normal flow of blood is disrupted. Being outside its channels (blood vessels), it pools and stagnates. As a result, the Qi of blood, the motive power, also stagnates, and obstruction occurs.

The concept of Qi is simple yet not simplistic. Fundamental aspects of Qi that concern us in trauma medicine are blood Qi flowing through vessels and **IE** (defensive) Qi, which permeates the body and occupies the interstitial space. When blood serum is interstitial, **IE** Qi is blocked. These blockages result in the accumulation of sui, water. In addition, the accumulation of water (edema) further blocks the flow of Qi interstitially and within the vessels. Physiologically, this places a strain on the kidneys and the heart, as well as the lymphatic system.

Trauma is not only from blows or falls, or cuts; obstruction may come from the environment: wind poisoning, cold poisoning, dampness, or heat accumulation.

These etiologies may combine heat-wind, cold-wind, damp-wind, damp-cold, and damp-heat. Proper treatment addresses these factors, adapting treatment procedures accordingly.   Local inflammation occurs when **IE** (protective) Qi, hot by nature, accumulates. **IE** (protective) Qi gathers not only because of obstruction caused by leakage of blood from its channels but because **IE** (protective) Qi is directed to the injury site to repair and energize the obstructed energies. When **IE** Qi is sufficient, the injured area is in the best position to self-correct and self-repair.

Treatment is to assist the system in reestablishing its internal equilibrium, so the myaku (meridian) Qi, **IE** (protective) Qi, and ketsu (blood) Qi can flow clearly. The energy blocked manifests as inflammation, pain, swelling, and dysfunction.

Modern medicine addresses body health with the Western model of cellular and tissue physiology and pathology; meridian medicine also concerns energy flow. If there is obstruction, especially for too long, then the blockage affects more than the injury site. The damage will occur by the buildup of energy in the area preceding the obstruction with depletion of energy beyond the blockage. Here we are looking at the flow of energy, which is not linear but spiral.

Preceding and beyond are terms relative to the direction of the flow of meridian energy and which aspect (yin/yang) of which meridian is affected because the meridians flow in different directions. In other words, distal/proximal or inferior/superior is determined by the nature of the meridian, not by an anatomical model.

According to the nature of the injury and its force, the bi syndrome will be as severe as the levels of energetics affected.

Physiologically, surface injuries obstruct the surface vascular system and skin; serious injuries affect fat, fascia, muscle and ligaments, tendons, bones, and internal organs. In addition, there are the surface meridians, tendomuscular meridians, main meridians (affecting organs), extraordinary meridians (affecting meridians), and, deeper still, the energy within the bones themselves.

Within the study of meridian energetics, we encounter these various layers or levels relating to the internal organs: skin - large intestine and lung; soft connective tissue – stomach and pancreas; tendons, muscles, and ligaments – gallbladder and liver; bone – kidney. We also encounter anatomical/meridian/organ relationships, such as index finger - large intestine, eye - liver, ankle – kidney, and so on.

Having evolved through martial arts, the essential practices of hands-on acute care techniques use the fingers and the heel of the hand. Use fingers, thumbs, and knuckles to affect care, as in shiatsu. Depending on the practitioner's skill, the injury's site, and nature, the pressure exerted may be more forceful ("deeper"), extended by rotation or pinching, or more focused by very directed force through the fingertip. The practitioner's proficiency in the hand Qi exercise further enhances the treatment.

Kappo resuscitation techniques extended beyond injuries received in martial arts training and Samurai warfare to different forms of trauma, such as drowning, heart attack, hypothermia, and other critical care situations. Kappo, in the context of our studies, means direct intervention in acute and chronic conditions to preserve life and enhance recovery and rehabilitation from acute and chronic traumatic conditions.

One technique in the kappo category that is neither anma, massage, nor shiatsu delivers a jolt to the body, provided primarily to the area of the back yu points along the side of the spine. The direction of the force is toward the base of the neck, Tokumyaku #14 (Daisui), the seventh cervical vertebrae. Deliver a jolt from two to six inches from the body using the heel of the hand, the thumb, or the knuckle of the middle finger, a tapping percussion technique. A variation is to use the ulnar aspect of a closed fist and perform a percussion technique. You may provide this with both hands unilaterally and bilaterally. Treatment is effective on the upper back, scapular region, and shoulders. This technique, termed katsu, is like the "obstructed airway" technique taught in first aid and CPR classes. The Heimlich maneuver, before it was termed "the Heimlich maneuver," is a kappo technique used for centuries for drowning, choking, and other breathing issues, including heart attack.

Shiatsu and anma treat soft tissue injuries, relax tendons, stimulate meridians, relieve cramps and spasms, relieve pain, promote circulation (Qi and blood), address stagnation and obstruction (thus reducing edema or swelling), and resolve facial and muscular adhesions.

These techniques are for acute conditions, developed "on the mat" in judo dojos. Therefore, they are most useful for fainting, convulsions, muscle cramps, fatigue, internal bleeding, and other acute situations.

Usually, the point of treatment is near or on the injury site. For example, a blow or blunt trauma injury to the kidney and lumbar region may cause internal bleeding, a general sense of bodily weakness, or mental disorientation. Treatment could be on lower Tai Yo #23 (Jinyu) using anma or shiatsu techniques. In this case, the provider would be standing over (straddling) the prone person and applying pressure to the injured site. If it is too painful, treat on the noninjured side until relief allows treatment on the damaged area.

MOXIBUSTION

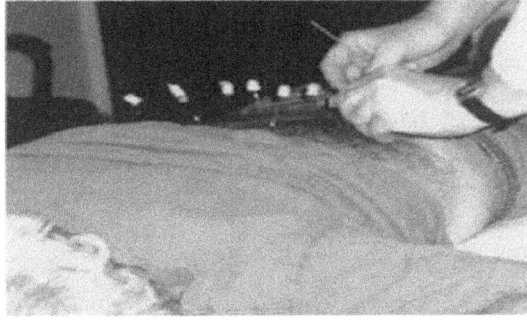

I do not presume to teach hari or kyu in this text. We have true experts in our midst now. Therefore, I have nothing to offer except to suggest that you never stop trying to improve your capacity. Concerning moxa, I respectfully point you toward the teachings and writings of Mizutani Junji Sensei.

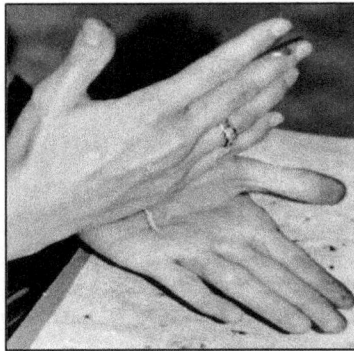

Moxa Therapy Shared by Nakazono Osensei

Moxibustion schools use these tsubo for all types of illness, providing direct moxa (okyu) regardless of pulse diagnosis, using abdominal and visual findings. Provide a treatment protocol of direct moxa, a half-rice grain size, one so* to these tsubos each treatment session. (*So is the term for an application of moxibustion in a treatment. There is the application of X # of so, commonly an uneven number, to a tsubo within a treatment.)

Tsubo treated in support of adult preventive care, using needle-moxa.

Lower Yo Mei (St) #36 (Ashi No Sanri),
Upper Yo Mei (LI) #4 (Gokoku),
Tokumyaku (GV) #4 (Meimon), Ninmyaku (CV) #12 (Chukan)

Magraine balls and indirect moxa, three to five so, are applicable:

Lower Tai Yo (Bl) #43 (Koko),
Lower Tai Yo (Bl) #20 (Hiyu),
Lower Yo Mei (St) #36 (Sanri),
Lower Sho Yo (GB) #25 (Keimon),
Lower Ketsu Yin (Lv) #13(Shomon), Lower Yo Mei (St) #25 (Tensu), **Treatment for all pediatric ailments:**
Tokumyaku (GV) #4 (Meimon),
Tokumyaku (GV) #12 (Shinchu),
Ninmyaku (CV) #9 (Suibun),
Lower Yo Mei (St) #25 (Tensu)

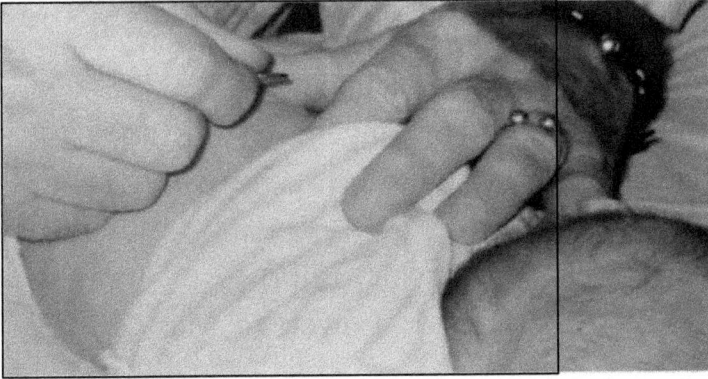

Moxa Treatment for Preventive Healthcare to Avoid Illness and Strengthen the Body

For treating those younger than thirty-two years, use needles, particularly with lower Tai Yo (Bl) #36 (Fubun), or you may cause an acid stomach. After age thirty-two, moxa is better. Direct moxa is the treatment of choice, but you can use the moxa stick. Be consistent with the points you choose. Be consistent with the time of the month, treat the same points, the same number of days, and the exact dosage. Treat three to eight days each month, five to eleven *so*. Direct moxa: use half rice size. After burning, press down on the skin, leaving the ash; burn the next one on top of the ash. With the first grain, moisten (traditionally with your saliva) to stick it to the skin. If you use all these points, only provide three to five *so* and only treat for three days. Be consistent. Taking those points each month improves blood circulation, enhances the strength of the cells, improves hormonal balance, awakens points and meridians, and maintains a healthy balance of meridians and tsubo.

Tokumyaku (GV) #12 (Shinchu)
Ninmyaku (CV) #4 (Kangen)
Lower Tai Yo (Bl) #22 (Sanshoyu) Lower Tai Yo (Bl) #36
(Fubun)
Lower Tai Yin (Sp) #9 (Inryoshin)
Lower Tai Yo (Bl) #13 (Haiyu) Lower Yo Mei (St) #25
(Tensu)

Long Life Moxa Therapy Treating lower Yo Mei (St) #36 (Ashi no Sanri) has a strong effect on the **(U)** dimension, Chu Myaku, the digestive system.

This protocol may cause hyperacidity or digestive issues in young adults. Therefore, you should not use it before age thirty-two. However, if the patient lacks Life Energy and is under thirty-two, you may use this protocol with caution. This procedure is a monthly eight-day treatment. Treat at the same time each month: the first day, your birth date, New Moon, or Full Moon. Choose a routine and follow it. Use direct moxa the size of one-half to one rice grain. Seek consistency in the size you use.

This treatment increases red and white blood cells, strongly affecting the heart and promoting longevity.

Traditional: Start on the left on a male and then go to the right; start on the right on a female and then go to the left.

Treat bilaterally.

Day	First Side	Second Side
1	9 so	8 so
2	10 so	9 so
3	11 so	11 so
4	11 so	10 so
5	9 so	10 so
6	9 so	9 so
7	9 so	8 so
8	8 so	8 so

Special Varicosity Treatment with Moxa

Varicosity is an oketsu condition and indicates weak vascular walls of a weak circulatory system. To shrink the surface veins, use stick moxa and slowly wave the moxa stick up and down the length of the vein(s) but not too close.

First is Hon-ji treatment; if there is discomfort after treatment, provide Hyo-ji treatment.

If you do the Hyo-ji treatment first, you may mask symptoms and get yourself lost.

HARI

The hands are the tools of healing. The acupuncture needle is a sacred extension of the practitioner's hand, dedicated to one master, balanced Qi. *"Regard the needle as the samurai regarded their weapon. It is a manifestation of your soul. It is an extension of your hand."* These words from Osensei need to be your commitment.

The spirit of the needle has been nearly lost, and it calls for renewal and rededication. The future of acupuncture relies on a return to past ways, a return to classic diagnostic methods, and the Neijing and Nanjing treatment rationales, united with the Kototama Principle.

My first needles were gold, employed to enhance/ho treatment, and silver to liberate/sha therapy. We sharpened and cleaned our needles after each treatment; they were our swords. As we used and honed them, they grew shorter and smaller. The "fire needle," high caliber surgical steel needle with which we provided kyu-hari therapy, could keep an edge (sharp point) with a whetstone for about 50 insertions. In 1979, we cleaned our gold and silver needles with alcohol; fire needles were autoclaved.

In the 1920s, Ken Sawada Sensei predicted the next primary concern for society's health would be protective Qi.

By the 1980s, HIV/AIDS brought about a significant alteration in the manufacture of acupuncture needles. Cheap, massproduced, disposable needles became the norm. Accordingly, dedicated acupuncture practitioners accepted the obligation to be even more seriously conscientious in the way and responsibilities of the needle. Through tanden-to-finger communication, a cheap, mass-produced needle can become an excellent tool in meridian therapy.

Reactions to hara, hari, and moxa treatment:
1. A yang condition feels stable with the conditions of the organs inside, and outside activity is hyper-normal and overactive. A yang reaction feels better internally and quickly begins showing signs of improvement. Described as being like a propelled arrow.

2. Kyo condition feels weak, like losing Life Energy. A yin reaction is an internal reaction: vomiting, nausea, a tired and dull feeling, headache, muscle, joint pain, loss of appetite, and sleep issues. It is like a roller coaster ride. These reactions will cease within twenty-four to thirty hours of treatment.

Restore Therapy

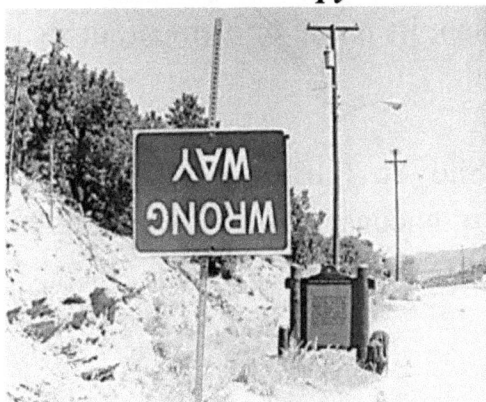

Inadequate or incorrect needling may cause the energy to flow in the opposite direction. It can occur with overtreating, misusing a point, treating the wrong meridian, or using a forbidden point. In other words, mistreatment by the practitioner. If you make such a mistake, the patient may have adverse reactions, such as diarrhea, sleeplessness, headache, fainting, pain, or paralysis. The energy is going in the wrong direction, and you need to change that. These techniques modify the energy flow created by improper needling techniques. These techniques are to "take back" the original condition to normalize the situation. These treatments are liberating (sha) techniques. Typically, with these techniques, you wait ten to twenty seconds before removing the needle or needles.

Basic considerations:
- Mistreat upper San Yin/San Yo— take back from under San Yin/San Yo.

- Mistreat lower San Yin/San Yo— take back from upper San Yin/San Yo.

Some forbidden points that produce specific problems address the same issues in the hands of a skilled practitioner.

Some schools and systems recommend using points on the mistreated meridian, its phase or element, or its back-yu point for Restore treatment.

Treating lower Sho Yo (GB) #21 (Kensei) may cause shock, lightheadedness, or unconsciousness. Treat St #36 (Sanli) and GB #34 (Yoryosen)

Concerning all tsubo on the abdomen:
If a needle touches blood vessels or shocks the energy current, it can cause pain and difficulty breathing. Treat the problematic point by planting needles 0.2 tsun-0.3 tsun below (distal); enhance/(ho) treatment, okibari. Address pain anywhere on the body caused by touching a blood vessel or shock to the myaku as you would for abdomen points.

If mistreatment causes fainting or paralysis, use a Restore point associated with the symptom.

Restore Treatment—Regions of the Body

Lower Abdomen (below the navel): Take back from under Sho Yo (GB) #43 (Kyokei).
Use okibari technique.

Lateral abdomen: location of lower Sho Yo and lower Yo Mei: Use points related to the mistreated meridian, that is, treat the same meridian or element.

Abdomen: Breaking or bending a needle occurs most often if the patient moves or the muscles contract. If the needle hurts the patient, treating lower Yo Mei (St) #26 (Gairyo) will calm it down. Provide Enhance/Ho treatment. Use okibari technique. Plant the needle toward the problematic needle.

Abdomen or Chest Area: Take points on the back opposite and parallel to the damaged area, especially the upper yu points and the scapula region. Use arm and leg points corresponding to the same meridian or same element principle.

Posterior or Medial Arm: Take upper Tai Yo (SI) #13 (Kyokuen) or lower Sho Yo (GB) #21 (Kensei), or lower Tai Yin (Sp) #6 (Saninko). Use okibari technique.

Back, Sacral Region: Take lower Tai Yo (Bl) #13 (Haiyu), lower Yo Mei (St) #36 (Sanli). Use okibari technique.
Medial Calf: If mistreatment is causing numbness or cramping, treat lower Sho Yo (GB) #36 (Gaikyu). Use okibari technique.
Posterior Calf: Treat lower Sho Yo (GB) #39 (Kensho) or lower Tai Yo (Bl) #60 (Konron). Use okibari technique.

Special Point: There is a point between the third and fourth toes at the joint of the tarsal bones. It has no name. In Japanese, it is mumei, which means "no name." You can use this point anytime the use of a point causes pain.

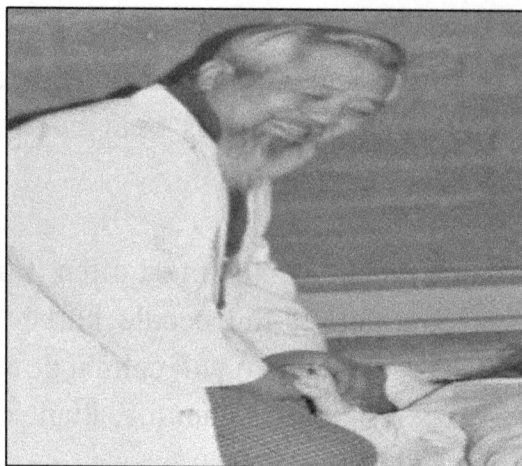

CHAPTER TEN

KOTOTAMA INOCHI PULSE

DIAGNOSIS

Life power echoes through the blood vessel.
  Pulse diagnosis is the basis of examination in meridian therapy.

I have drawn on the teachings of Masahilo M. Nakazono's comprehensive understanding of the Kototama Sound Principle in the Five Element mother pattern (A, I, E, O, U) within tai kyoku. He brought the six aspects of Life Energy within San in/San yo (Tai Yin, Sho Yin, Ketsu Yin, Tai Yo, Sho Yo, Yo Mei) and the seventeen hidden gods, the vital life force, diagnostically into relevance.

In addition to the pulses, Osensei thoroughly examined the patient's forms, signs, and expressed dimensions. He studied every facet and factor—bun shin (listening diagnosis), mon shin (questioning diagnosis), bo shin (looking diagnosis), and setsu shin (touching diagnosis)—to confirm a conclusion and always from the vantage point of the Kototama Principle. As stated, since antiquity, 'wrong diagnosis, wrong treatment' or 'the treatment lies within the diagnosis.

'What is the Kototama Principle vantage point? It concerns focusing on the unfolding of the universal creative process, consciousness, and the unfolding of life.

First, there is "the big bang" manifesting tai kyoku (tai chi), stillness and movement, yin and yang, sounds of life awakening (A), life will (I), life power (E), life continuation (O), life formation (U). The sounds are the elements of life in form. Go Gyo, Five Elements, present as the universe's expression of itself and first manifest as wave and particle, as vibrations seeking to create an ear to hear, a voice to speak.

First, there is one, tai kyoku.
From one comes two, yin/yang.
From two comes five, Go Gyo
From five comes all that manifests. Everything manifests from A I E O U Five dimensions of Life Energy within one.

Apriori - the inherent properties of the Universe's self- formation: universal lifeforce of being (A), universal life- will-tobe (I), universal life-power-to-be (E), universal life continuance-of-being (O), universal life-form-of being (U).

Aposteriori - the finite properties of life's self-formation: sensations of life, spiritual (WA), presence and expression of life and self-being (WI), empowerment of life, self- essence (WE), retention of life, memory (WO); structure of life, physical being (WU).

In ancient times, in China, the emphasis was on the importance of pulse diagnosis; Japanese practitioners focused on abdomen diagnosis. After the turn of the twentieth century, political factions almost destroyed all traditional medicine practices in China.
Herbal medicine, an oral tradition needing neither texts nor tools, endured. Pulse diagnosis and hands-on treatment, including acupuncture, went underground. In Japan, pulse diagnosis experienced a rebirth, with many studies focused on combining pulse and abdomen in diagnosis and treatment. Masahilo M. Nakazono combined pulse diagnosis, meridian therapy with Kototama Sound practice and studies.

Serious attention to the pulses is becoming a lost art. Pulse diagnosis, referred to as the "radical way," takes years of training and can only be accomplished in a clinical setting between a student and an experienced senior. Traditional medicine has become academic; it is not clinical but studied in classrooms and postgraduate workshops. Learning by guidance from an individual with years of experience has increasingly become inaccessible. There are books about pulses, but actual pulses are only in living beings. The learning of pulses occurs in the clinic, on a living being. The senior guiding the junior in a clinical setting is "the way of the pulses." It takes years to begin to grasp. Individuals who can quiet their minds and egos and remain in the state of "student" forever may learn the way. That is what it takes.

There are traditional doctors of oriental medicine who only use pulses in conjunction with other diagnostic methods. They do not understand pulses. However, do not debate such issues. Do not be arrogant, and do not be foolish. The best use of looking, listening, and questioning diagnosis is in touching diagnosis. Practitioners well-skilled in pulse diagnosis discover a wealth of information about their patients through this method alone. Pulse reading is the most critical aspect of diagnosis, revealing much. Understanding the pulse tells the condition of Life Energy within the system.

The pulses are at the center. Diagnose by abdomen; also check the pulses. Diagnose by Akabane method; also examine the pulses. Treat with handwork; check the pulses. Always treat the abdomen with handwork. Always check the pulse and obtain instant feedback on the practitioner's influence on the patient. Spiritual Axis (Ling Shu) stated, "Must check the pulses before, during and after needling, to know, to grasp the Life Energy of that patient, their energetic condition and make the correct differentiation."

"Every time you plant a needle or give one so of moxa, check all the pulses again, noting the changes that have occurred. You must be serious this way. To attain the highest capacity for pulse diagnosis, you should not read the pulse in a dualistic way, with the sense that, 'I am now seeing the patient.' Read the pulses as your life rhythm and vibration, becoming entirely one with the patient. You will slowly improve that way and find the right sense for this pulse diagnosis. It is a very delicate matter, and it is not easy to read them correctly. You cannot do it by concentrating only halfway; you need to be really, completely concentrating."

Masahilo M. Nakazono, class notes, 1978

Diagnosis by pulse is a subtle art, far more than any other diagnostic procedure. It requires tremendous attentiveness, experience, patience, humility, and arrogance to acquire the sensitivity necessary to grasp it. One of our professional ancestors,

Wang Shu-he, wrote: "The mechanisms of the pulse are fine and subtle, and the pulse images are difficult to differentiate." He stated verbal definitions of pulse conditions are easy to memorize, but "it is difficult for the fingers to distinguish them." (*The Pulse Classic*)

"In Japan," Nakazono Osensei told his first formal class of students of

Kototama Life Medicine. "It is held that when a person has read the pulses of ten people a day for ten years, that person <u>may</u> earn the title of a beginner." It is like that. I began my study of the pulses with Nakazono Osensei in 1977. I am serious; I am just a beginner. There is so much more to comprehend.

"A practitioner who, after years of experience, develops expertise in reading the pulse deserves the utmost respect."
                    Dr. Stepan T. Chang, Internal Arts Magazine

Proficiency in pulse diagnosis enables the practitioner to determine the most minute energy imbalance in the body at the time of diagnosis and the past causes of disease, which lead to the current imbalance. Being able to read past imbalances as a prelude to current conditions means the practitioner can also predict future inequities based on current conditions. For this reason, the practitioner well-practiced in pulse diagnosis can predict the future concerning health issues and is, therefore, a specialist in preventive healthcare and maintenance.

When the Inochi practitioner reads the pulses and conducts additional diagnostic work, the focus is the energy itseWe are not merely treating the human body; we are addressing the original multifaceted strength of the body, assisting that energy to rebalance itself so that it may continue toward fulfilling its unique potential. The pulses express the energy by which a cell, an organ, or an entire system exists. We diagnose and treat the life behind cells, organs, systems, and the energy that creates and maintains these systems. Sickness manifests in the weakest space in the system.

Our studies concern vibratory energy at or before the cellular level. We do not treat symptoms of organ dysfunction; we treat that which is before organs come into being. This vibratory energy is tai kyoku or tai chi. Fu Hsi, the author of the I Ching, defined tai kyoku as "absolute void point." The pulses of tai kyoku are the space where we observe the individual's energy. The pulses present the energy for which there are organs. There is a heart, kidneys, and bowels; the energy that creates and sustains these organs reveals itself through the pulses. The energy in creating and maintaining the large intestine existed at, perhaps before, conception. Without that energy, there would be no large intestine. Subsequent removal of parts, the energy is still palpable. People with their gall bladder removed remain with a gall bladder meridian and pulse, which may be jitsu or kyo. We are diagnosing and treating this energy.

Through physics, we experience that overlaying a complementary waveform results in a new waveform without destroying the integrity of the original waveform.

All life forms are a new waveform resulting from fundamental complementary Life Energy waves overlapping each other. The ancient Greeks labeled the original waveforms *apriori* (without form, selfevident) and the resulting new form *aposteriori* (having appearance, observable). Modern physics now speaks of implicate and explicate, implied, and unfolding. Nakazono Osensei used the terms apriori— formless, that which comes before— and aposteriori— form, that which comes later—as the division taking place with the Big Bang, the moment of the birth of the universe, the space dividing finite and infinite.

At the time of conception, Life Energy (I) and capacity (E) of the new form (U) exist. The development is incomplete; its life energy is complete. The life form reaches full emergence through the cycle of formation, birth, youth, adult, elder, death, and dissolution.

The Seventeen Pulses of Kototama Natural Life Therapy

The method of reading pulses, developed in Asia, is the most significant contribution to diagnostic procedures. There are seven pulses at each wrist (including the six basic), a bilateral pulse in the neck, and an abdominal pulse. These "seventeen hidden gods" state and reflect Life Energy.

The radial pulse biomedical practitioners monitor is the location of the seven pulses read at the wrist. It is the Life Pulse, Chu Myaku in traditional medicine, considered a source of vital information concerning the quality of Qi and other life issues. It is engaged bilaterally because of the often distinctly different manifestations of unbalanced Qi from one side to the other.

Roku-bu-jio-yi, Sun-Kan-Shaku-bu-joi, "both hands-six pulses." **Twelve pulses**.

Chu Myaku, Life Pulse, middle pulse. The Life Pulse expresses the U dimension, physical function, and nutritional Qi as fundamental to Life Energy. It is that person's individual Life Energy itself you are reading. It indicates if its imbalance is slight, moderate, or severe; it will tell if this individual has a long, medium, or short life; this pulse will reveal much to one who is quiet, still, and listening outside of time without thought or anticipation. **One pulse**

Go gyo hara, Five Element abdominal pulse. **One pulse**

Do/so, normal/noisy pulse. **One pulse**

Jingei myaku, fu/zo jitsu pulse. **One pulse**

So-yin, personal pulse. The So-Yin pulse is the most crucial. It is an aspect of the person's primary pulse condition. It belongs to the basic constitution inherited from the parents—the Jingei pulse aids in understanding the So-Yin pulse. If we do not know about or do not consider this pulse, we will sometimes make the wrong diagnosis. This pulse is not easy to grasp in early treatments. As treatments continue, the patient's ill feelings and condition disappear, yet the pulses are not entirely balanced; something in the pulse is slightly off. It may be that the sickness has not yet healed completely, or it might be this patient's original pulse condition. One cannot be cavalier about pulse diagnosis. If you cannot see what condition exists, you may keep trying to balance them, and treatment goes on for a long time. If it is the patient's so-yin pulse, the therapist will have worked and suffered unnecessarily, and the patient will have gone through unnecessary trouble, expense, and overtreatment. We must know about this matter. It is much more evident through the jingei diagnosis—**One pulse**.

BEGINNING OF PULSE DIAGNOSIS

"It is important to understand that when you make a diagnosis, the way our ancestors taught it, you must be in the void— without knowing anything. Do not diagnose from experience or knowledge; always have an innocent mind. You need this sense for all four ways of diagnosis, but it is vital for pulse diagnosis. Do not think about yin/yang, the Five Element principle, or the patient's previous condition. Always read the pulses as if it were the first time."

Osensei

Pulse diagnosis is attuning oneself to another so that one pulse exists. *"Read the pulse."* Yes, sniff the pulse, feel the pulse, grab the pulse, and hear the pulse. Osensei tasted the pulses through his fingertips. Be the pulse.

Traditionally, one would see the doctor in the morning unless severely ill. Old documents suggested taking the pulses in the early morning because this is energetically the calmest time of the day— blood circulates more regularly and calmly. The idea is that the patient and the physician are calm and relaxed when taking the pulses, using Sakai Sensei's hand Qi centering technique and Kototama breath exercise. You read the pulses from your tanden and supply calm by your presence.

Protocol in pulse reading should include having the patient wait at least five minutes upon arrival, allowing them to arrive to begin attuning to the energy in the practitioner's space. If making a house call, wait ten minutes after arrival before beginning energy work. What is the hurry? Post- treatment is also essential because Qi requires twelve hours to circulate through the meridians. Post-treatment should include rest.

Ideally, the patient should not be on medications, alcohol, or drugs, nor should you.

Osensei instructed patients receiving treatments only to take lifesustaining prescriptions and to discontinue all other medications, supplements, and herbs while undergoing treatment. He opposed such influences on the pulse dynamic and any form of therapeutic intervention not grounded in Qi.

Take pulses with the patient lying on their back (supine). Stand erect with your knees relaxed and spaced about two fists width apart. The patient needs to be relaxed, and the physician needs to be unhurried.

Traditionally, you start with the patient's left side. Tradition is a reference point, not a theology. You pick left or right. Get centered and clear. Extend the patient's hand slightly so that the pulse area is flat. Sit or stand at a 90-degree angle to the patient. Have no thoughts, no expectations; "hear" the pulse from Qi of tanden.

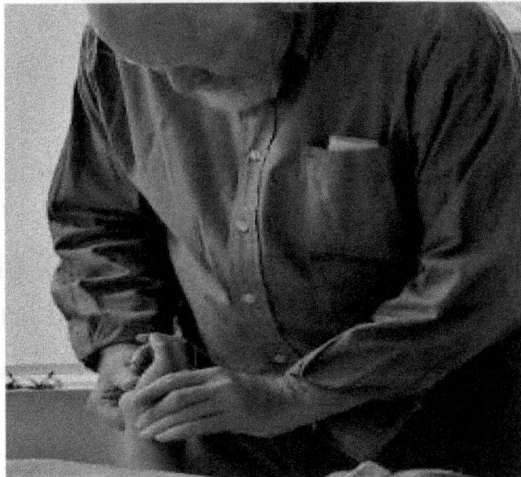

Physical Presence of Roko-bu-jio Pulses.

Sunko (**Sun**) is on the wrist at Upper Tai Yin (Lu) #9 (Taien)- 6 bu distal of Kan.

Kanjo (**Kan**) is at the styloid process at Upper Tai Yin (Lu) #8 (Keikyo). This pulse is slightly more robust due to the styloid process; do not confuse it with a Jitsu condition.

Shaku-chu (**Shaku**) is seven bu proximal to Kan on Upper Tai Yin (Lu) #7 (Rekketsu).

The pulse consists of three components: <u>position</u>, <u>speed,</u> and <u>form,</u> and each component has two alternatives: floating/sinking, fast/slow, and choppy/slippery. The further back in history, the simpler the descriptions of pulses. Over time, various voices added more adjectives, and more translators added more interpretations. There are now at least twenty-four qualities of pulses identified. They are subtle distinctions from each other, refined statements about the primary condition. The primary condition is pulse disorder, kyo, or jitsu. (below)

Each location has three positions:

Floating Pulse/Fu Myaku - Superficial position: belongs to the yang meridians and discloses yang dysfunctions and the external part of the body. If insulted, (IE) Qi/protective Qi is disturbed. Place the fingers lightly on the radial artery with the ball or tip of each finger, touching the skin to feel the pulse—Decipher from Sun to Shaku with the ball of the finger lightly on the skin. Begin checking with the index finger. Three fingers can read the condition at once. Feel it under the skin but at the surface of the body. Do not use your thumb to exert pressure. Instead, go to the middle position, Chu Myaku (IE); press slightly and slowly release. If the pulse disappears before the pressure is fully released, the pulse is kyo (-). If the pulse is over-abundant, it will remain after the pressure is lessened and recognized as jitsu (+).

Middle Pulse/Chu Myaku - Middle position: Life current pulse. Place fingers on the radial artery with slight pressure. Gently sense the pulse between the skin and the superficial muscles. Here you are communicating with Chu Myaku (I/E), the Life Pulse. Chu Myaku is the pulse of the physical life (U) dimension and contains vital information. From here, examine yin/yang, kyo/jitsu, aspects of so-yin pulse, and longevity. It is the space of nutrition, physical maintenance, and perseverance. In some traditions, Chu Myaku, Life Pulse, is called the 'Stomach Pulse,' in some traditions. In Kototama, Chu Myaku reflects (I/E) in (U), Life-Will's power in form.

Symptoms relating to **Chu Myaku** pulse qualities:

Sudden (Tense) Indicates cold in the body.
Relaxed Indicates fever in the body.
Big Indicates abundant Qi, less blood.
Small Indicates Qi and blood are both deficient.
Sliding Indicates Yang Qi is very abundant, inconsequential fever

Stagnating   Stagnation of Qi
current, insufficient
blood, slight cold;
there may be blood,
swelling, discharge,
or possibly a tumor.

Sinking Pulse/Zo Myaku - The deep position conveys the conditions of the yin meridians, showing yin dysfunctions and the internal body. When insulted, sei Qi/internal healing Qi is affected; read from Shaku to Sun. Place the fingers on the radial artery and exert steady pressure. Feel the pulse within the deep muscle in the radial pulse. Press deeply to feel the pulse. Begin checking with the ring finger. Start at the middle position, Chu Myaku, slowly applying pressure, press to the bone. Read one finger at a time. If the pulse stops before reaching the bone, it is weak, kyo (-). If it is still present after touching the bone, it is too strong, jitsu (+).

So-Myaku, the Six Basic Pulse Conditions

Initially, four actions were observed within the wrist pulse that differentiated the state of Qi: Floating, Sinking (noted above), Fast, and Slow. Fast/Saku Myaku is rapid, with six or more beats per breath cycle. Saku indicates fever, overheating, showing yang-type illness. Reducing the heat with Liberate (sha) treatment is necessary. Use needles, moxibustion, handwork, herbs, poultices, compresses, or whatever achieves your goal. If needling, plant deep quickly, out fast, and do not close. If using moxa to liberate, use fewer points and more heat. Slow/Chi Myaku presents a slow pulse, less than four-five pulse beats per breath cycle. Chi Myaku is a Yin disorder, indicating a decrease in heat. Enhance (Ho) treatment with moxibustion, handwork, herbs, soaks, and compresses. Gently assist a systemic return of warmth. Plant shallow needles or provide Enhance (Ho) moxibustion.

Later, Jitsu/full-excessive and Kyo/empty-deficient distinctions became established. Kyo denotes weakness, an imbalance indicative of stagnation of Life Energy. Sickness contributes to the depletion of Life Energy. The patient may or may not feel weak or sick but will present an unwell feeling. The practitioner must be sensitive to the weakness in the patient. Jitsu indicates force, full of energy, an imbalance indicative of inflammation. The patient feels strong because the illness's energy is manifesting its strength. The patient may feel it as Life Energy; it is not. As the jitsu condition continues unaddressed, the energy dissipates, and the system begins losing its vital force. Chu Myaku, the middle pulse, may reveal a death pulse.

Accessing the Information in the Pulse
There are five necessities when focusing on the pulse.

1st - Observe the pulse-as-a whole.

2nd - Experience the "spirit" of the pulse.

3rd - Recognize the voice of the pulse.,

4th - Feel the strength of the pulse.

5th - Sense the condition of the meridian through the pulse.

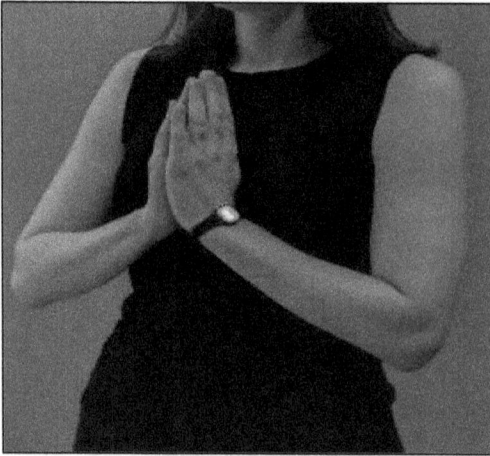

To feel the pulse, you and your patient are relaxed and breathing fully.

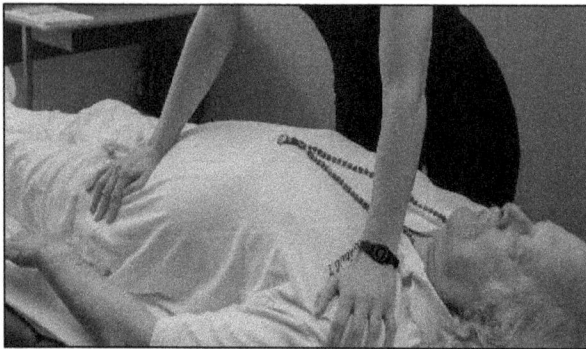

Find the imbalances in the four corners, the shoulders, and the hips. Note everything. Position yourself perpendicular to your supine partner. Reach across and cup the shoulder with the heel of your hand on the brachial pulse at the anterior aspect of the joint; simultaneously, cup the hip and inguinal junction with the heel of the other hand - on the femoral pulse at the groin. Be in your tanden with equal attention to both brachial and femoral pulses. Maintain a consistent presence, stay quiet, and wait until both pulses have consistent rhythm and force. Do this from your tanden; use no strength. Focus and feel what is going on there. Feel the pulse? What is its vibrational power? Are the brachial and femoral pulses synchronized? Note everything. Release from the tanden and press down the thigh to the knee several times. Do not press on the kneecap. Repeat on the side closest to you; then perform this contact diagonally. You invite the brachial and femoral pulse to synchronize on both sides of the body, diagonally and in-line, termed "balancing the four directions." Encounter imbalances; correct with pressure. This procedure should relax your patient; therefore, pressure with no strength and hold the pressure for only ten seconds.

Have no thoughts or expectations when taking pulses. Do not push; go there. Do not look at notes or records of previous treatments before taking the pulses. You must have an empty mind. Be in the present.

Nakayima. Be. Now.Here. Breathe into tanden and exhale SUUUUUU. Osensei reminds us: "If pulses are read based on memory, knowledge can never be acquired, only more memory."

When taking pulses, do not apply pressure; politely go there. Start by placing your middle finger on the ridge of the styloid process of the radius, index finger at the wrist crease toward the thumb, and ring finger proximal to and equally distant from the middle finger. Then, pressing firmly but without pressure, feel Chu Myaku, the middle pulse, the life power pulse. You can read yin or yang from here. To train in pulse diagnosis, one must practice hand Qi exercise daily. The more you practice, the more powerful you might become.

If the pulse feels too weak or too strong, hold for fifty pulsations, and observe. What changes? A healthy person's heart pulsates four to five times per breath, count the patient's breathing. The pulse rate considered normal in Inochi Medicine is sixty-four to seventy-six. Less than fifty beats per minute is slow unless the person is a professional athlete; above eighty beats per minute in an adult is usually too fast.

The beginning moments of pulse diagnosis involve ascertaining akashi, evidence. Positioned on the patient's left side, place your non-dominant hand on the sternum. Examine breath and palpitations. Gently move your hand to the lung bo point area and check lung Qi. Smoothly move below the sternum to examine spleen/stomach Qi. There should be a pulse around the navel—mid-line. If it is too strong, it is a jitsu condition; too weak, kyo. If too strong, consider stomach/spleen jitsu. To distinguish the stomach/spleen requires checking the wrist spleen pulse. Then move your hand to the lower abdomen to examine the lower heater (ka sho) and kidney Qi. Next, assess liver Qi along the abdomen below the ribs. Finally, observe heart Qi and heart palpitations in the area below the left nipple, at the apex of the heart. A pulse slightly discernible is a sign of good health; not discernable is a sign of ill-health; a pounding pulse is a sign of an extremely critical condition, perhaps a "death pulse."

Diagnosis means to realize which myaku are losing balance. Myaku translates as pulse and includes meridians (Kei myaku and Ryaku myaku), blood vessels, the circuitry of Qi energy, and consciousness flowing through the body. So- myaku is the primary pulse situation. Pulse diagnosis is where we diagnose the meridians and evaluate meridian energy. The pulses are alive.

Diagnosing meridians includes comprehending how each of the meridians affects the others and understanding their relationships. Is the loss of balance due to deficiency, kyo? Or is the loss due to excess, jitsu? By the pulses, which meridian is the cause of imbalance? Touch along the meridian to learn which points react. Find the tsubo on that meridian that will have the most influence.

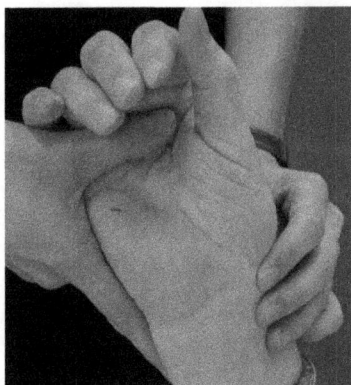

"When the Qi of the five zo circulates fifty times, there is a balance."

The pulse at the Sun position reveals the balance between organs. When the pulses are balanced to each other, and the pulse does not stop within fifty beats, that is, not irregular or does not skip a heartbeat; it indicates the zo organs are adequate.

When the Sun pulse stops once in forty beats, there is a lack of Qi in one of the zo organs.

When the Sun pulse stops once in thirty beats, there is a lack of Qi in two of the zo organs.

When the Sun pulse stops once in twenty beats, this indicates a lack of Qi in three zo organs.

When the Sun pulse stops once in ten beats, there is a lack of Sei Qi in four zo organs.

When the Sun pulse stops once in less than ten beats, this is a severe condition indicating the patient is dying.

If a pulse is weak, touch along the meridian to learn which points react.

Wang Shu-he stated, "If a deep pulse is considered a hidden one, the protocol and treatment will never be in the right line (meridian); if a moderate pulse is regarded as a slow one, a crisis may crop up instantly." He further noted that different pulse conditions might manifest simultaneously, and various illnesses and symptoms may exhibit the same type of pulse. "Life hangs on the practice of medicine," he stated. "Even the most excellent of physicians … had to deliberate before they arrived at a correct diagnosis." The treatment is within the diagnosis: wrong diagnosis, wrong treatment.

The masters throughout the ages have provided various undertakings and interpretations of the *Neijing* and *Nanjing* and have taught many ways and descriptions of the pulses.

Wang Shu-he said, "The writings left by our predecessors are pregnant with such far-reaching imports that only a few in later generations have been able to practice them, and the arcane transmitted in the old classics are too abstruse and enigmatic to be divulged. Therefore, later, students have been kept in the dark about the ins and outs (of the study of the pulses)."

The Pulse Classic.

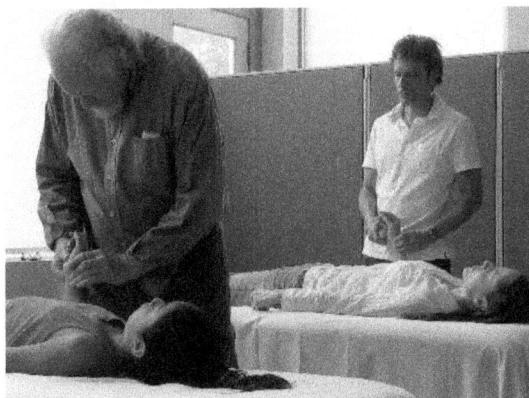

Take each Pulse individually; they are clearer to read. Always compare the pulses, fu to fu, zo to zo.

Nakazono Osensei provided these four historical pulse interpretations in *The Law and Therapy of Natural Life* (1981)

1) <u>Chu Myaku - Nine Ways Pulse</u>. Shows challenging conditions of disease. For these pulses, do not pay attention to the fu or zo pulse; feel Chu Myaku, the middle pulse.

Cho: Long, extending beyond the sun-kan-shaku line at both ends. It indicates fever and yang (overexpansion) poison in the organs. It is difficult for the patient to lie down or sit up.

Tan: Feels like a grain of rice, small and short. It is so short it is perceived only on the kan pulse. Exceedingly difficult to heal. It suggests upper abdomen pain.

Kyo: A floating and large pulse that is soft and slow. It indicates a kyo condition of yin meridians and fever.

Saku: Beats over five times per breath. It indicates a fever.

Ketsu: A little slow and slows even more from time to time. Indicates a jitsu condition of the yin meridian; blood and Qi cannot flow.

Dai: Irregular pulse that regularly stops every ten, fifteen, or twenty beats.

The patient is losing Life Energy. The energy is weak.

Ro: A big, long pulse indicates a jitsu condition of yin meridian energy. It feels solid and unending. Yin energy cannot change over to yang.

Yang meridian has completely lost balance with yin; there is no life. The body swells, and the breath is rough.

Do: Shows only on the Kan position, at the middle level. It is like a small, rolling bean. Indicates cramping of hands and legs, and all physical strength is weak. Also, it indicates blood in urine or stools or cannot control urine.

Sai: Appears in the middle (Kan) position of the pulse. Indicates loss of blood energy; physical strength is weak, making the body thinner.

2) <u>Pulse of Sichi-Hyo - Seven Upper (Fu) Pulses.</u> These surface pulses usually show an acute condition. The pulse is on the surface; the sickness is in the fu meridians. **Fu:** Feels movement floating on the surface of the pulse. It indicates a jingei/sunko upper condition.

Kyo: Like a scallion, there is nothing inside when pressed. It indicates loss of blood.

Katsu: Smooth undulating, like running a finger along a string of beads. Indicates kyo condition, a lack of strength.

Jitsu: Same feeling as katsu, like a string of beads, but this condition feels stronger. It shows when there is vomiting with mucus.

Gen: Like the taut string of a bow. It indicates lower Ketsu Yin/lower Sho Yo and upper abdomen problems.

Kin: Thinner, like a twisted silken thread, pulling and hard. It indicates fever, pain, and swelling or tumors.

Ko: Large, full, strong jitsu. It usually indicates a yang-jitsu condition and high fever.

3) The Pulse of Hachi-Li - Eight Bottom (Zo) Pulses. It usually shows chronic conditions. The sickness is in the zo meridians.

Bi: Feeble and tiny pulse. When firmly pressed, it disappears. It indicates a deficiency of Qi and blood energy. The patient may feel chilled or is quickly chilled.

Chin: Sinking but has strength; yin meridian jitsu condition. A sunko condition.

Kuan: Slow and slightly floating, usually indicating a slow pulse.

Shoku: Means not going forward smoothly ("shy to go ahead"). not smooth. The energy gets stuck and has difficulty coming out. The pulse is small and difficult to feel. It is continuous but not fluid, a kyo condition, and may indicate a contraction in blood circulation. This pulse is commonplace in bleeding situations and diarrhea. **Chi:** Pulses less than three times per breath indicate body heat deficiency.

Faku: Felt at the bone, at the bottom. It is difficult to read and is usually caused by overheating (heat poison), but it is of brief duration and will change to a jitsu pulse.

Nan: Floating and feels like soft cotton to the touch; there is no strength. It indicates a kyo condition of Qi and blood.

Jiaku: Sinking and like touching soft cotton, feeble. It indicates a total loss of strength.

4: Yellow Emperor: Six Kinds of Pulses. Read at the Shaku position.

Smooth - most natural. Nothing to change. Provide moderate teate.

Sudden or tense - feels hurried, may be slow or fast, indicating cold in the body. Treatment: Proceed deeply; leave needles until the fever comes out. Wait for the heat to surface. If the body is cold, it compensates for a fever somewhere.

Big - a physical sense of the pulse. Shows deficient Qi and excess blood. Treat to liberate (sha) Qi, but do not do sha ketsu treatment.

Small – a physical sense of the pulse. It shows Qi and blood are both deficient. Correct through nutrition. An example: Lower Tai Yin is kyo, providing a slightly sweet taste in foods is appropriate. Hari (needle) treatment is too powerful for this condition; handwork may even be too intense.

Sliding - it feels like your finger is sliding across glass. Indicates abundant yang Qi and slight fever. Enhance (ho) treatment, following the meridian flow, and close the hole immediately.

Stagnating— it feels as if the pulse is vibrating under your finger. Indicates Qi stagnation, insufficient blood, cold, or a tumor. The stagnating condition means stagnation of Qi current; it is sluggish, therefore, stimulate. You need to Enhance (Ho) and Liberate (Sha) to bring about the proper flow of Qi. The stagnating pulse is very much affected by teate.

Check one pulse at a time; is it clear? robust? drained? It is best to compare the individual pulse with the other single pulses. Check, compare the bilateral Chu Myaku pulses and identify the side more substantial. Is the right side stronger on a female? Or is the left stronger on her? Check the left side on a male. Which side is stronger? Are they equal? Traditionally, if a male's pulse is more energetic on the right hand or a female's pulse is stronger on the left, the condition is more chronic and will be slower in response to healing. This issue needs study.

If you are unsure about the pulse, stay there, and hold that position. The pulses are alive. Take your time. You are determining the actual condition. You are either correct or wrong. Some practitioners will read the pulses for an hour before starting or acting on a diagnosis.

The kan position, middle position/middle finger, may feel slightly more substantial because of proximity to the styloid process and is not to be confused as a jitsu condition.

All pulses are equal, of equal value, and of the same strength. If a pulse is unhealthy, touch along its meridian, and detect reactions. In the event of trauma in any form, the complete system will react. The injury will immediately show out as jitsu, the reaction of protective Qi. Even though the entire system responds to injury, as a practical matter, if one meridian is jitsu, its paired meridian will be kyo. Remember, you are always dealing with the entire system.

A regular pulse has a medium frequency of four to five beats per breath in one cycle of breathing, inhalation- exhalation, with a steady rhythm, even and equal force, termed a 'do' pulse. A 'do' pulse in a healthy person presents sixteen to eighteen cycles per minute. The biomedical normal pulse range is sixty to seventy-eight times per minute. A pulse rate below fifty is bradycardia; it is considered too slow. Athletic people often have a regular rate below fifty.

A pulse rate above eighty is termed tachycardia and is considered too fast in a resting adult. A rapid heart rate shows the energy has become overabundant in the upper meridians, a 'so' ("noisy") pulse. A 'so' condition manifests as a noisy, rushing, buzzing pulse. The 'so' situation typically presents a heart rate over eighty but, focus on whether the state is noisy; a heart rate can be below eighty and be a 'so' condition. 'So' may indicate high blood pressure, asthma, facial or head inflammation, energy stuck in the upper body, or chronic disease.

Death Pulse

When the twelve wrist pulses present strong, rigid, and identical: termed "a cancer vibration," a death pulse and said to be irreversible, with the prognosis of "no hope." With cancer, there is a unique vibration in the pulse. When all twelve wrist pulses show the death pulse, and you also get this cancer vibration, there is no hope. The death pulse is not absolute, but this situation could be. I have observed such a pulse condition change and improve. It is tricky; you should always try your best. The life-will (I), while expressing information in the pulses, including the Death Pulse, knows its own time. We should not interpret such findings as unfavorable or even as likely. Treat the best you can and watch life unfold.

Seven Death Pulses (according to the Somon of the Neijing)

Jaku-Taku	Like a bird pecking, stopping, then pecking again.
Okuru	Like water dripping down from the roof.
Dan-Seki	Like hitting a hard place, like a stone.
Ai-Saku	Like strands of rope unraveling
Gyo-Sh	Like fish's tailing moving back and forth.
Ka-Yu	Like a frog coming up to the surface of a pond, hovering, and then quietly disappearing below.
Fu-Futsu	Like bubbling, hot water.

The Inochi Pulse Pattern

The study of the Kototama Principle led to the Kototama Inochi pulse pattern that identifies the left wrist pulse as Sun-Liver, KanSpleen, and Shaku-Kidney and the right wrist pulse as Sun-Heart, Kan-Lung, and Shaku-Shimpo. My focused research on pulses began in 1982. I started a clinical investigation of this pulse arrangement in 1984 and offered my findings to Nakazono Osensei in 1986. I have used this pulse arrangement consistently since 1986 and have taught my students this diagnosis since 1988. This way is designated Inochi Pulse Diagnosis.

INOCHI PULSE DIAGNOSIS
MYAKU POSITIONS

SUNKO (sun)   KANJO (kan)   SHAKU-CHU (shaku)

Right Wrist – So Pulses

Right Fu: Upper Tai Yo   Yo Mei   Sho Yo

I   E   YI

Chu Myaku

Right Zo: Upper Sho Yin   Tai Yin   Ketsu Yin

WI   WE   WYI

Left Wrist – Do Pulses

Left Fu: Lower Sho Yo   Yo Mei   Tai Yo

A   U   O

Chu Myaku

Left Zo: Lower Ketsu Yin   Tai Yin   Sho

Yin   WA   WU   WO

The locations of Sun-Kan-Shaku are traditional. Interpretations of information provided at Sun-Kan-Shaku positions:

The left wrist reveals the energy of the Lower Meridians.

Left Sun position: **A** dimension – Strong pulse when jingei/sunko 1x under condition - Life Purification – "liver meridian" - a deep pulse, slow to resolve, suggests San Yin/San Yo involvement with (**Y**) dimension (Shimpo meridian). Mother of (**I**) dimension.

Left Kan position: **U** dimension – Strong pulse when jingei/sunko 3x under condition - Life Nutrition – "spleen meridian" – a deep pulse, slow to resolve, indicates San Yin/San Yo involvement with (**E**) dimension (lung meridian). If there is predominant strength in the distal aspect of this pulse, consider the pancreas. Mother of (**A**) dimension.

Left Shaku position: (**O**) dimension – Strong pulse when jingei/sunko 2x under condition; life fluids – "kidney meridian" – A deep pulse indicates San Yin/San Yo involvement with (**I**) dimension (heart meridian). Mother of (**U**) dimension.

The right wrist reveals the energy of the Upper Meridians:

Right Sun position: (**I**) dimension – Strong pulse when jingei/sunko 2x upper condition - Life Blood – "heart meridian" – Deep pulse shows a chronic condition with(**O**) dimension involvement, San Yin/San Yo. If there is predominant strength in the central aspect of this pulse, consider the anterior thorax. If there is predominant strength in the lateral aspect of this pulse, consider the posterior thorax. If there is predominant strength in the proximal aspect of this pulse, consider the diaphragm, especially in the region of CV #14, Heart Bo tsubo. Mother of (**E**) dimension.

<u>Right Kan position</u>: (**E***)* dimension – Strong pulse with jingei/sunko 3x upper condition - Life Breath – "lung meridian' - Deep pulse indicates (**U***)* dimension involvement, San Yin/San Yo. Mother of (**Y***)* dimension, Shimpo.

<u>Right Shaku position</u>: *(***Y***)* dimension – life enhancement – "Shimpo Meridian" – jingei/sunko 1x upper condition. A deep pulse indicates (**A**) dimension involvement, San Yin/San Yo. Mother of (**O**) dimension.

INOCHI PULSE DIAGNOSIS

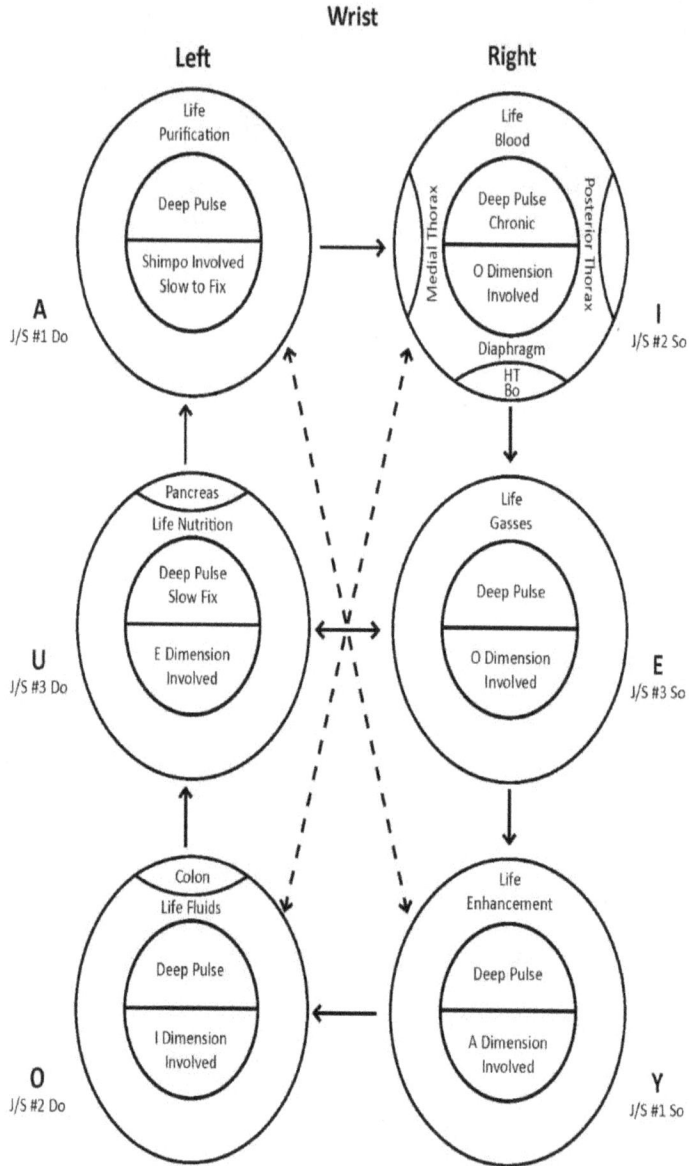

Wrist

Left   Right

A
J/S #1 Do

Life
Purification

Deep Pulse

Shimpo Involved
Slow to Fix

I
J/S #2 So

Life
Blood

Medial Thorax

Deep Pulse
Chronic

O Dimension
Involved

Posterior Thorax

Diaphragm
HT
Bo

U
J/S #3 Do

Pancreas

Life Nutrition

Deep Pulse
Slow Fix

E Dimension
Involved

E
J/S #3 So

Life
Gasses

Deep Pulse

O Dimension
Involved

O
J/S #2 Do

Colon

Life Fluids

Deep Pulse

I Dimension
Involved

Y
J/S #1 So

Life
Enhancement

Deep Pulse

A Dimension
Involved

JINGEI/SUNKO PULSE DIAGNOSIS

Jingei, Lower Yo Mei (St) #9, is on the carotid artery.
Sunko, Upper Tai Yin (Lu) #9 (Taien), on the radial artery.

There are many types and ways of secrets. Some of the best-kept secrets are right in front of us. When Osensei taught us jingei diagnosis in 1980, he treated it as a secret. He swore his students to secrecy in deference and respect of Dr. Dokei Ogura (1899-1983) (also Ogura Dokei, Doeki Ogura, Do Kei Ogura). The man who undertook a twenty-year exploration of ancient writings to understand and revive this diagnostic procedure.

Nakazono Osensei regarded the physician as a priest and warrior, "cut from the same cloth" and guided by a code of conduct comparable to samurai or knights of the Round Table. It concerns honor without defining the term. From that place of honor, I have refrained from publicly speaking of jingei diagnosis, honor to Dr. Dokei Ogura. Recognition and gratitude to Masahilo Nakazono Osensei for teaching jingei diagnosis to North America and sharing it with us.

It was February 1980. We were in our eighteenth month of total saturation: Tai kyoku, yin/yang, myaku, ryoku-bu-jio- yi pulse diagnosis, Go Gyo principles, so sei, sokoku, abdominal diagnosis, moxibustion, teate, Akabane, diet, kyo, jitsu, ho, and sha. It was the end of class. Osensei looked at his eighteen serious students.

"Are you willing to die to further the medicine?" he asked. He restated his question, "Are you willing to die for information that would improve diagnostic skills?" He smiled at our confused look. Had we not been dying all along? Then, he laughed, "I do have a serious question. Are you willing to take a blood oath, a life oath, that you will honor the secrecy of a specific diagnostic method? That you will keep it strictly to yourself? Would you make a sacred oath to that effect?" Individually and collectively, we answered, *"Yes."* "Good, then go practice misogi and come back tomorrow dressed in your very best," he directed.

The next day, we arrived at the dojo dressed appropriately, having fasted, bathed, and practiced breathing exercises and Kototama Sounds. Osensei explained the ritual he was about to perform and informed us that afterward, we would need to puncture a finger and use a drop of our blood as the seal to our promise not to reveal this sacred trust, this new diagnostic piece of information. Did we agree? *"Yes."*

He began beautifully chanting the Fifty Kototama sounds in the Sugaso, Kanagi, and Futonrito orders and Shinto noritos, thanking ancestors of the past, present, and future for the gift of sharing in the wisdom of healing. When he finished, he told us we did not have to draw blood; he was checking to see how serious we were. Then, he began to teach us the way of jingei diagnosis.

This pulse diagnostic method, designated "jingei," read on the carotid artery at lower Yo Mei (St) #9 (Jingei*)*. The Yellow Emperor's Canon, Huang Di Neijing, discusses these practices. Taking the pulse at the carotid artery seems to predate the pulse diagnosis at the radial artery.

Such had been the situation concerning the jingei diagnosis. It is traceable to the Neijing, Ling Shu, and Su Wen; the Nanjing; and the text, Full Use of 14 Meridians, written sometime between the twelfth and fourteenth centuries, but it fell out of usage for about seven hundred years

Dr. Ogura began publishing his research in the Ido-Nippon- Sha Journal, which is how Nakazono Osensei learned of it. After that, Osensei started to use it in his clinical practice, sharing his thoughts and discoveries with the Ido-Nippon- Sha Journal and Dr. Ogura.

Dr. Ogura palpated the pulses with the patient seated. He used the thumb and index finger of one hand to palpate the carotid artery on both sides and palpated the radial artery with the index, middle, and ring fingers of his other hand.

Dr. Ogura described the ideal jingei and sunko pulses as having three features:

First, the jingei and sunko pulses should have an even ratio of force and volume.

Second, they should correlate with the seasons, as expressed in chapter 48 of the Spiritual Axis (Ling Shu). That is, during spring and summer, the jingei pulse is slightly more significant as it is in the yang aspect of the body. Conversely, during fall and winter, sunko should be slightly fuller, not more significant, than jingei.

Third, there should be no irregular force, volume, or arrival rate shifts between jingei and sunko pulses.

The kyo (deficiency) and jitsu (excess) conditions of ``the twelve main meridians (keiraku) are assessed through the ryoku-bu jio pulse diagnosis, clarified, and confirmed by the jingei diagnosis.

The twelve main meridians (Kei ryaku) result from San Yin/San Yo, the three aspects of yin/yang.

Lower	Myaku	Upper
Spleen	Tai (large)Yin	Lung
Kidney	Sho (small) Yin	Heart
Liver	Ketsu (middle) Yin	Shimpo
Bladder	Tai (large) Yo	Small Intestine
Gall Bladder	Sho (small) Yo	Sansho
Stomach	Yo Mei (lesser)	Lg. Int.

Roku Bu Jio wrist pulse informs concerning the energetic activity of each specific meridian. Jingei pulse ascertains the dominant jitsu meridian and indicates where to focus treatment in the San Yin/San Yo (three yin/three yang) relationship.

Nakazono Osensei used the jingei diagnosis on every patient for several years. All the background research and information had come from data obtained by treating Japanese people in Japan. Osensei was treating North American patients. He found Dr. Ogura's distinction between the pulses slightly different from his own.

Through his study of Kototama, Osensei discovered a more precise way to understand, interpret, and treat the meridian pulses; through jingei diagnosis, he uncovered the means to guide students to diagnose and treat Life Energy effectively. His study of the Kototama Principle led to the Futonorito alignment of Go Gyo. In the jingei diagnostic pattern, he saw the symmetrical arrangement of this paradigm. Once he grasped the jingei diagnosis within this context, he opened the Kototama Institute to teach Kototama life-centric meridian therapy.

As he explained to his students, "Jingei diagnosis completes the view that the Kototama Principle lies at the root of meridian therapy and allows a complete treatment protocol within the framework of Kototama
Five Element Medicine and the San Yin/San Yo meridian relationship."
Osensei could see that his theory of the Kototama Five Element paradigm, Futonorito order, was supported through the jingei diagnosis.

Jingei diagnosis is in addition to the ryokobu-jio-yi pulse diagnosis and guides the study of San Yin/San Yo (three yin/three yang). The kyo (deficient) and jitsu (excess) conditions of the Kei ryaku are evaluated through the ryoku-bu-jio pulse and clarified and verified in the jingei diagnosis.

DIAGNOSTIC TECHNIQUE

Exert the same pressure at Jingei and Sunko positions and compare the pulses for tempo, thickness, taste, rhythm, activity, and warmth. What are their comparative strengths? Note that the radial pulse is smaller, so the carotid will always feel bigger. The Jingei/Sunko Pulse diagnosis is not about size but strength and vibration. We are diagnosing energetics, not quantity. Check and compare bilateral wrist pulses and take the more energetic pulse. Check and compare bilateral neck pulse and choose the more energetic vibration.

Compare these two pulses.

Use the comparative qualities for purposes of prognosis. The disorder will remain chronic and challenging to resolve if both pulses are firm and slippery. If the pulse is soft in arriving, the problem will be solved readily.

> The jingei/sunko pulse reveals the most jitsu, the most "disordered" meridian. Nakazono
>
> Osensei researched Dr. Ogura's understanding of jingei, verified his considerations, and arrived at this pattern "disordered" meridian pattern. **Jingei**

1) Jingei 1x is Sho Yo myaku jitsu when the jingei and sunko pulses are comparatively the same, with jingei being one to one-and a-half times stronger than the jingei pulse. (Dr. Ogura classified this as two times stronger.)

2) Jingei 2x is Tai Yo myaku jitsu when the jingei pulse is twice stronger and more active than the sunko pulse. (Dr. Ogura classified this three times stronger.)

3) Jingei 3x is Yo Mei myaku jitsu when the jingei pulse is three times stronger than the sunko pulse. (Dr. Ogura classified this four times stronger.)

4) Jingei 4x is found when the jingei pulse is four times stronger than the sunko pulse; yang is so extremely jitsu it cannot communicate with yin. "Yang is not rooted." The pulse is large and speedy. The yang energy is flooding and refuses to synchronize with the yin energy; the outside and inside cannot synchronize a severe condition. It is correctable. (Dr. Ogura classified this as five times stronger.)

Sunko

1) Sunko 1x is Ketsu Yin myaku jitsu when the sunko pulse is one to one-and-a-half times stronger than the jingei pulse. (Dr. Ogura classified this as two times stronger.)

2) Sunko 2x is Sho Yin myaku jitsu when the sunko pulse is two times stronger than the jingei pulse. (Dr. Ogura classified this as three times stronger.)

3) Sunko 3x is Tai Yin myaku jitsu when the sunko pulse is three times stronger than the jingei pulse. (Dr. Ogura classified this as four times stronger.)

4) Sunko 4x when the sunko pulse is four times stronger than the jingei pulse; yin is closing so firmly, it cannot communicate with, is unable

to synchronize with, yang. (Dr. Ogura classified this as five times stronger.) It is large and fast. Indicates all the yin pulses are jitsu. "Yin is being closed." It cannot or will not turn over to yang. Osensei said, "It is like the energy of a stone." Another expression is "closing down inside." It is considered a death pulse. It is considered a condition that cannot heal, and the patient "is obliged to die." Jingei and sunko (myaku) pulses are more than four times normal strength— "Heaven and earth obstructed," meaning that both sides, yin and yang, mutually resisting synchronization.

Upper/Under Conditions

When the diagnostic condition of the patient concerns the lower meridians of the body, this is a do condition. 'Do' condition means there is a regular pulse. However, it is not loud, urgent, or fast. The heart rate is usually between sixty to seventy-eight beats per minute and termed an "under" condition, such as "jingei 1x under," "sunko 2x under," etc.

When the diagnosis relates to the upper meridians of the body, this is a 'so' condition. 'So' is not a regular pulse. It is noisy, loud, urgent, pounding, buzzing, rushing, and fast. The heart rate is usually over eighty beats per minute, five to six beats per breath - an "upper" condition, i.e., "jingei 1x upper," "sunko 3x upper," etc. An upper state indicates Qi is stuck in the upper meridians. It could signify hypertension, pulmonary issues, fever, cancer, acute pediatric situations, or trauma. A 'so' condition usually has a heart rate over eighty, but the focus is not the rate per se; it is the noisiness. A person could have a heart rate of seventy-two, which could be a 'so' condition; conversely, one could have a rate of eighty-four, which is not a 'so' condition.

You must listen.

A healthy person manifests as an under ('do') condition. Many imbalances manifest as an under ('do') condition. Everyone in health will show a jingei 1x, 2x, or 3x 'do' state. "1, 2, 3" do not indicate progression, just phenomena. From birth, we are jingei 1x, 2x, or 3x 'do'. We present diagnostic conditions when we are out of balance. Diet, emotions, ecology, and DNA influence our energetic patterns. When treatment successfully addresses the regaining of equilibrium of our original condition, we will show our original dynamic state through the jingei (see "So-Yin Pulse").

Jingei - Jitsu in Fu
Under/Do

Jingei 1x indicates GB is Jitsu

Jingei 2x indicates Bl is Jitsu

Jingei 3x indicates St is Jitsu

Jingei 4x, rare, Enhance (Ho) all under zo myaku.

Upper/So

Jingei 1x indicates Sansho is Jitsu

Jingei 2x indicates SI is jitsu.

Jingei 3x indicates LI is Jitsu

Jingei 4x indicates extreme condition, can fix; enhance all zo myaku.

Sunko - Jitsu in Zo
Under/Do

Sunko 1x indicates Lv is jitsu

Sunko 2x indicates Kd is jitsu

Sunko 3x indicates Sp is jitsu

Sunko 4x, prognosis very weak, enhance (Ho) all under fu myaku

Upper/So

Sunko 1x indicates Shimpo is jitsu

Sunko 2x indicates Ht is jitsu.

Sunko 3x indicates Lu is jitsu

Sunko 4x is a death pulse; enhance all the fu myaku. Do your best.

Reminders:

> In a sunko diagnosis, at least three zo pulses will show jitsu.

> You must exert the same pressure at the jingei and sunko positions.

> Compare pulses for tempo, thickness, rhythm, activity, and taste. If both pulses are firm and slippery, the imbalance will remain chronic and challenging to resolve. If the pulses are soft, the imbalance will resolve quickly.

Anatomically, the radial artery is smaller than the carotid artery. Therefore, the carotid artery will feel more prominent, but we are not observing anatomy.

Check bilateral wrist pulses and choose the stronger. Check bilateral neck pulse and determine the strength. Compare these two pulses.

Check the wrist pulses and determine which is more substantial. When a male has stronger pulses on the right side or a woman on the left side, the condition may be more chronic and respond slower. Maybe not. All for your serious studies.

Treatment protocol of jingei/sunko diagnosis, employing treatment principles of enhance (ho)/ liberate (sha) when treating so sei or San Yin/San Yo relationships: Jingei or Sunko 1x—may treat once a day. Jingei or Sunko 2x—may treat once every two days. Jingei or Sunko 3x— may treat twice a day.

Consider the following points therapeutically with the diagnosis of:

Jingei 1x (TH & GB): Lower Yo Mei (St) #25 (Tensu)

Jingei 2x (SI &Bl): Lower Sho Yin (Kd) #12 (Daikaku)

Jingei 3x (LI & St): Lower Yo Mei (St) #27 (Daiko)

Sunko 1x (HC & Lv): Lower Sho Yo (GB) #24 (Jitsugetsu)

Sunko 2x (Ht & Kd): Lower Sho Yin (Kd) #16 (Koyu)

Sunko 3x (Lu & Sp): Lower Ketsu Yin (Lv) #13 (Shomon)

I have found that when the wrist pulse is 'do,' bilaterally equal, and not a sunko condition, the patient responds to very gentle treatment. Enhance (ho) and liberate (sha) therapy to the Gen (Source) Points or a singular relevant point.

CONCLUSION

<u>Treatment:</u> Having determined the meridian with the most kyo condition through studying and comparing Roko-bu-jio and jingei pulses and deciding whether to treat the So Sei (mother-child) or San Yin/San Yo (six-channel system) relationship by incorporating looking, listening, questioning, and touching diagnosis, I treat with hari, kyu, and teate, from *SU*. The Nakazono-Kototama lineage teaches how to correct the pulses with handwork as the entry into acupuncture before teaching needling. Therefore, handwork is always a component of treatment. Sometimes, it is the only treatment. The first phase of treatment is to enhance (ho) and liberate (sha). The second is teate and kappo from head to toe, with attention to the abdomen. Next, teate and kappo to the back with extra care where you encounter stagnation, also on the regions that correspond to the primary pulse condition and the Go Gyo findings on the abdomen. If Enhance and Liberate reach completion on the patient's back, then teate commences on the back. I may utilize sotai techniques and provide specific kappo and muscle-skeletal stretches. I may provide "Tamatouch," the finger-thumb touch treatment of the extraordinary meridians. I will check the pulse multi- times during treatment; it is the only way I can monitor my treatment in "real time." If any jitsu pulses remain, I will do additional teate to the abdomen to take down the jitsu condition. I know the session is complete when the pulses are 80 percent in balance. I let the patient know we are finished by saying "thank you." The treatment is complete within twenty to thirty-five minutes.

There are a few practitioners who have studied this way. They have climbed out of the box to achieve outstanding results. I wish you well in your studies.

Appendix Osensei's 108 Warrior-Priests

A Beginning School of Natural Life Medicine Masahilo M. Nakazono Osensei, Founder

Opening Ceremony
September 1978

"I offer you my congratulations upon entering this course. You have all decided to study here for a minimum of two years, and I would like to talk to you about your reasons for doing so. You may think it resulted from a personal decision, and that is true. But there is also a deeper reason, something at the bottom of each of you, a larger sense that motivated your choice. This is a manifestation of the human Life-Will.

"All human beings, consciously or unconsciously, are guided by the action of the Life-Will which lies at the bottom of every decision made. This activity is the same for everyone, but when it manifests as aposteriori life, as our present human capacity, physical and spiritual, each displays individual and different desires. Because of this, each one of us must search to discover where our most significant interests lie and where we can most seriously put all of one's energy. When we find our authentic way and can concentrate on that path, that is the moment we become a missionary.

"If I were to speak religiously, I would say you were sent here by Heaven to do this work as God's angel. The real meaning behind such words as Heaven or God has to do with the pure substance of the human life-will itself. The Kototama Principle shows it to us as the motive vibration of the sound of the *I* dimension. The human Life-Will, *I*, acting in judgment, is **_E_**. This action of **_I-E_** creates the human body, without error, in its physical form as aposteriori life. It realizes the capabilities of each physical life until that life is finished.

"The aposteriori action of everyone is guided by the highest judgment of the Life-Will **_I-E_**. As I said, there is only one **_I-E_**, which is the same at the bottom of all human beings. Each one's aposteriori capacity, however, is different from the other. It can never be the same, just as our appearance is not the same or as someone with superior strength, an excellent memory, or a sharp intuition that always makes the right judgments. Each one has a different strength or ability and to a different degree.

"As you study, you will gradually realize why this is so. I shall not discuss it today, but I passionately believe that our highest judgment, **_I-E_** guides us in the best way possible according to each one's aposteriori capacity. It watches and judges which is the best way to use this person and, from the bottom of us, tells us the right way to go. The guidance of **_I-E_** comes out as an individual desire in our head, such as, 'I want to study this or that; I want to go this way; this subject interests me,' etc.

"For this reason, all of you made an individual decision to take this course. That means you are in the process of finding your path and mission, and going this way will help you see it more clearly. It will also make you more useful to serve in the development of human civilization. That is why you decided to enroll in this course; at the bottom, you decided to realize your mission this way. Slowly, as you continue the path, you will see this more clearly. As this school's textbook title indicates, this course is the study and practice of the law of human, natural life and its aposteriori physical body. The healing of sickness means restoring the body's proper balance. The basic premise of healing then belongs to the Kototama Principle. Thousands of years ago, our ancestors found the law of the activity of the Life-Will and its highest judgment *I-E*; created this principle and hid it from society about five or six thousand years ago. By the end of World War II, knowledge emerged. This matter is outside the scope of our study, but the real meaning of that disastrous war was for the Kototama Principle to return to us. Hardly anyone can see the great purpose behind the cause of this war. Slowly, you will understand its meaning yourself.

"Anyway, the essence of the Kototama Principle is the life-will of humanity, of *I* and the activity of judgment, *I-E*. The activity of aposteriori capacity *I-E,* can be seen and grasped by the spiritual action of human capacity, *A*. by the spiritual action of human capacity's spiritual action *A*. This *IE-A* is symbolized by three colors, red for *I*, white for *E,* and blue for *A,* which are also the colors of the American flag. The

The Republic of the United States is a collection of people who represent all the world's countries. And it raises a flag of red, white, and blue. This means it stands for the total desire, the unconscious will, of all the world's nations. It is the will to search this way, and the flag is an unconscious symbol of where the collective wishes to go.

"The fifty stars also have their symbolic meaning. The star means the scientific-material civilization. Fifty is the number of perfection or completion. The number of stars cannot become more than fifty. If we can see its real significance inside the symbol, the flag stands for the American people's life-will that is being unconsciously expressed.

There is only one life-will, the life-will of the universe. It is the same Life-Will and Life-Power at the bottom of all humanity. It acts from its highest judgment, creating the universal This is *I-E*, red and white. Try to find the truth of that reality and see it with your aposteriori human capacity. Only human beings try to see the law of the universe and its creation. This capacity is *A*, blue. The real meaning of the American flag is this nation's unconscious will, and the method of its search is through science, as symbolized in the stars. This nation's mission is the perfection of the actual material civilization.

"The human seed has kept the memory of the ancient times and already knows that the spiritual way of searching leads to the final truth of the Kototama Principle; there is no need to search any further in that direction. Only the scientific way of searching is necessary. Japan holds the spiritual truth handed down through the generations. The United States, as a conglomerate of all the nations of the world in cooperation, is trying to find the truth scientifically and will bring this search to perfection very soon. The people of these two countries have the same mission, but on either side of it, front and back, the work is separated this way.

"When I clearly understood this, I left Europe and came here. I am doing my best to awaken the spiritual memory of the Kototama Principle in my body, the memory of a thousand years in my traditional blood. From there, I compare actual civilization with the principle and give my best critical commentary to hasten its development. And then, you will remember the scientific study of the past five thousand years and compare it to my explanation so you can re-study it, look at actual civilization from this perspective, and be sure of it in yourself.

"I decided to give all my energy in the service of the perfecting of the spiritual and physical civilization. Having made this resolve, I feel strongly confident in my mission. All of you here must do the same as me and hold your inner confidence in your mission for perfecting civilization. I am asking you to awaken your missionary sense and to feel as I do.

"To demonstrate our dedication to that higher purpose, as taking an oath to oneself from this moment on, we will sing our national anthem. I will sing the Japanese national song, 'Kimigayo,' but first, I must explain it. During World War II, the Japanese nation was led by national militarism; the meaning of "*Kimigayo*" was perverted into a song that was only about the Emperor. From childhood, it was taught this way; even today, the Japanese people believe it to be so. That is why the Socialist and Communist parties are against singing that song. They fear it might inspire militarism again.

"We must read back the real meaning of "*Kimigayo*" according to the life principle of the Kototama fifty sounds to see what it says. *KI*-*MI* means one who has manifested with human capacity; it is a name used between people. *GA* is of, and *YO* is the world, generations, or epoch. The true meaning of "*Kimigayo*" includes the total meaning of the human world, civilization, and generations. It was never meant for only one person. It is an ancient poem from an unknown time that says humankind should continue a thousand generations, eight thousand generations; as a tiny stone becomes a great rock, as the rock becomes covered with moss, should civilization, the life of humankind, be so permanent. It is a prayer to praise and celebrate our everlasting life for the Japanese people and all humanity.

"So today, here-now, as an oath to serve all people, I shall chant '*Kimigayo.*' After that, as a promise to be true to your mission, you shall sing '*The Star-Spangled Banner.*' With that, we will conclude today's ceremony. Whatever intellectual understanding you may have of your anthem – you feel funny about singing it – you must remember that the flag symbolizes this nation's serious mission. I am asking you to sing this song to awaken from the bottom of yourself and heed the root desire of your life's voice."

First Graduation - May 1980

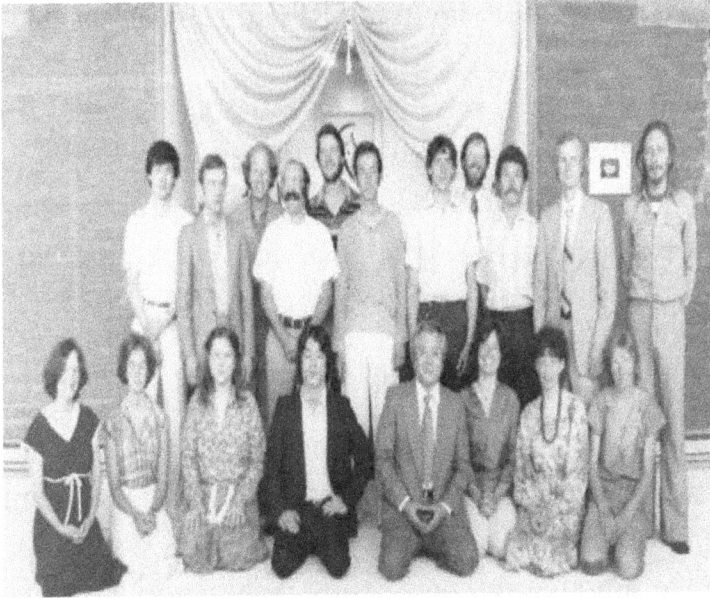

Masahilo Mikoto Nakazono Osensei
Katsuharu Kazumichi Nakazono Sensei

**Masahilo M. Nakazono Osensei Ceremony for the
Completion of the Initial Two Years of Study**
May 1980

"I have just now given you a certificate stating you have completed two years of study. It is not a diploma. Please understand that the school cannot give you a diploma without passing the practical examination. From my heart, I feel profound respect for your strong determination and challenging work during the past two years. Despite all kinds of difficulties, you were able to stick to your resolve to finish your studies. Now I am sending you out into society as specialists of natural medicine, equipped with the necessary basic knowledge and technique and more evolved

225

personality that is required. You are the first of the students to finish this course. It is a moment in my life of great honor because I am confident you will be doing great and helpful work for society "It is from now that the time and place for your actual study awaits you. You must not be afraid, and you should not be lazy. You must hold on to your serious spirit and courage more strongly than you have these past two years. You must go ahead, perfecting the way of your mission as I explained on the first day of class,

"At the same time, as you continue to search the way of natural medicine, you must not forget to keep a meek mind. You must always be new – a beginner – in here-now. Keeping this mentality is the most important thing to help you grow and develop. You must continue to practice self- reflection. When you have lost this humble mind, you should know you cannot grow and progress further than that level.

"I have already made diplomas for you, but that is for the future. I will watch you and make sure about the improvement of your capacity. Until I can feel completely satisfied, I will keep them with me in the hope you can return at the earliest possible time to receive them from me.

"I believe that I have already finished telling you what I have to say in class. You must remember all of it and recognize yourself as a missionary for perfecting the medical side of this civilization. You must continue, taking one step after another, with a sure and steady step. To express our gratitude and happiness for this day, to renew your vow for your future to be true to your substance of (*I*), to thank all the ancestors who, from the beginning, gave their divine love – for all these reasons, we have this ceremony.

"After the ceremony, I will sing '*Kimigayo*,' the song of permanent blessing for all humanity, just as we did at the first ceremony. Then you will sing again the 'National Anthem' – the song that says truth and freedom for humanity will prevail; it is the way that is permanent and everlasting and will never die. With that, we will finish today's ceremony."

**Masahilo Mikoto Nakazono Osensei
Last Graduation
Last Graduation - June 1985**

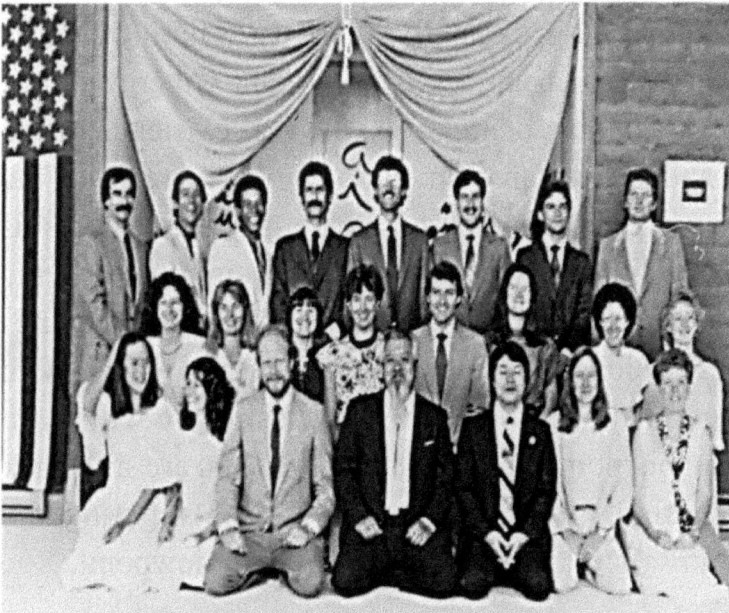

**Masahilo Mikoto Nakazono Osensei
Katsuharu Kazumichi Nakazono Sensei
Thomas E. Duckworth, Doctoral Candidate**

"Dear Students,

"For the Kototama practicant, all situations, whether 'good' or 'bad,' are all matters of phenomena. The subject, the self, exists, and therefore all kinds of phenomena will manifest. If there is no self to recognize them, these phenomena cannot appear. You must grasp this and ensure that you stand on this viewpoint. If our self is incomplete, then 'bad' situations are automatically created.

"If our judgment is based upon the knowledge of our lower dimensions, **A** or **O** dimensions, automatically from these viewpoints, we will divide the phenomenological world into 'good' and 'bad." However, in the dimension of the final truth, there are five dimensions of energy with concentrating activity and five dimensions of energy with expanding activity. This activity is recognized by the **IE** dimension acting with eight father rhythms. This is the source of human beings. It is the real existence of the universal center and, at the same time, the whole existence of the real source of our self. It is not possible to separate it; it is absolutely one. **I-WI** is the seer, the self, and simultaneous the object seen. If we cannot grasp this meaning, everything becomes relative, as in the division of yin and yang, subject and object. With this viewpoint, automatically by our will or desire, we will try to change and control phenomena to fit our wishes. You are still stuck in the lower dimension's world. Therefore, you are suffering and will continue to do so until you can get out of that viewpoint.

"The Kototama Principle is the absolute truth for yourself, but you should not force others into understanding. The time hasn't arrived yet for people to understand, and to try to force it becomes violence. Using force and power is the way of Amatsu Kanagi and Sugaso Principles but is not the way of Amatsu Futonorito.

"Try to throw out the content of your present knowledge, including your knowledge of the Kototama Principle. Your beliefs are the total content of your present O dimension; that is your entire property now. Throwing it out means dying to your present self. After you throw out the complete contents of your knowledge, absolutely nothing exists. That dimension is the door to the Garden of Eden; it is the first step toward the Kototama Principle. Jesus spoke of this as being born again, Christians talk of the Messiah's return, and Buddhists speak of Buddha awakening from a million-year sleep. These are all symbolic words left to us by our ancestors and are hints toward the final truth.

"So please read this letter carefully, reflect, and release yourself so you will be completely free. If you are nothing, you can never force another person. Everything exists in you; therefore, you can automatically realize and accept everything as it is. If you judge phenomena as 'good' or 'bad,' you will restrict yourself, and this will cause you difficulty. That is all. All my love to you.

Sincerely,
M.M. Nakazono

Graduates

1980

Beatrice Blake, Brian Brigham, Susan
Brigham, Thomas Duckworth, Charles Hollobaugh,
David Kelly, Sharon M. Nakazono, Sarai Saporta,
Robert Shijtaku, Hank Skrypeck, Silvi Solomon,
Paul Sowanick, Sondra Spies, Lou Talento,
Link Tate, Gary Vendemia, Steven Weiser,
Glenn Wilcox

1981

Stuart Bernstein, Phyllis Bonder, Maky Erdley,
Donald Goldstein, Greg Gorman, Martha Iwaski,
Anthony Kaluta, Kristie Kellerhouse, Kim Krull,
Richard Rosenbaum.

1982

Stanley Baker, Elizabeth Berringer, Guy Best,
Chris Butler, August Coulson, Joanne Dwyer,
Jody Erickson, Mitchell Gillman, Linda Hubbard,
Stanley Hubbard, Katherine Johnson, Randi Larson,
Gary Ludewig, Lola Moonfrog, Lisa O'Maley,
Dean Phillips, Jannika Reed, Christine Saunders,
Bunzo Takamatsu, Skye Taylor, Mateel Todd,
Richard Van Steenis, Maurizia Sanin

1983

Ted Annenberg, Hans Asmussen, Laurie Broslow,
Sidney Clifton, Susie Dean, Charles Draper,
Bobby Duckworth, Jean Meiss, Jeffery Nicholson,
Jan Phetteplace, Turtle Pratt, Glynda Ratliff, Paul Sonia,
Susanna Stewart, Valerie Talento, Hugh Wheir

1984

Elizabeth Allen, Ed Antkowiak, Kit Antonietti,
Pearl Brown, Jamie Campbell,
Christine Dukeminier, Jerry Dukeminier,
Ann Fiedler Cocolovo, David Goldman,
Martin Goldman, Walt Lucas, Oliver
McCrary, Roberto McEntee, John Poff,
Neal Sirwinski, Jeannie Smith,
Yahe Solomon, Arthur Teubner, Loni Yien

1985

Joseph Breslin, Melody, Karen Carpenter Day,
Denise Chevrefilis, Angelique Cook-Wilcox,
Nancy Crothers, Richard De Felice, Fiquet Hanna,
Leah Fineberg, Imetai Henderson, David Long,
Isis Lum Abbott, Glenn Moyer, Sharon Orbach,
Paul Pitetti, Michael Polera, Charles Quinn, Cathy Riggs,
Lenny Socolov, Jennie Thill, Ann Millikin, Jean Claude Taverner

GLOSSARY

Abdomen: The condition of the physical abdomen is a strong statement of the person's general health. The lower abdomen contains the small intestine, the appendix, the large intestine, reproductive organs, and the bladder; the upper abdomen includes the stomach, spleen, pancreas, liver, gall bladder, small intestine, and large intestine.

Albi: Taro root recipe consisting of 50 percent taro root flour, 40 percent wheat (glutinous) flour, 10 percent grated ginger root, plus enough water to form a very thick paste.

Ampuku: Abdominal massage developed as a profession in Japan several hundred years ago.

Anma: (push-pull) Traditional Japanese massage. The traditional method, ko ho anma, involves stretching, rotating, squeezing, pressure, rubbing, and kneading to stimulate vital energy. The functional reliability of physical systems sedated with pressure (an), normalized by rubbing (ma), rubbing/pressing, firm but gentle, and moderate. Use the palm or fingers/thumb to stimulate blood circulation directly, release stagnated blood in skin and muscle, and address all circulatory congestion, tension, and stiffness. Specialized treatment is on the floor; the modern method is on a table for relaxation.

Aposteriori: (from the later) From the perspective of Kototama studies, aposteriori is what exists in form. The expression of the sounds gives them a form that defines them as aposteriori, finite.

Apriori: (from the earlier) From the perspective of Kototama studies, apriori is what exists before form, infinite.

Ashi San Li (St #36): A significant point for longevity and strong legs. During the Edo period (1603-1867), the Manpei family, from the province of Mikawa, developed a protocol using Lower Yo Mei (St) #36 for strength and longevity.

Body Fluid: Sweat, urine, saliva, tears, and secretions. There are two types: Yang is lucid and thin and spreads through the skin and muscles; it warms, nourishes, and moistens the sensory membranes and the excretory orifices. Yin is turbid and thick or viscous; it lubricates the joint and tones and moistens the brain and the body's inner organs. Collectively, fluids are termed blood. Yin: blood; yang: Qi.

Burdock Root: A Japanese vegetable, gobo. It is a cooked root vegetable and pickled (fermented) condiment. This Eurasian plant species is a sunflower/daisy family biennial. It contains chemicals active against bacteria and inflammation. (This is how Osensei was able to ascertain that my daughter did not have appendicitis. Her symptoms did not change when she consumed burdock juice which directly affects appendicitis) A "blood purifier," used as an antibacterial, increases urine flow, reduces fever, and addresses colds and bladder infections. It treats cancer, anorexia, stomach and intestinal issues, joint pain, gout, diabetes, acne, psoriasis, high blood pressure, arteriosclerosis, liver disease, and appendix inflammation/non-ruptured appendicitis. Apply a paste or tincture directly on acne and minor skin irritations.

Chinetsukyo: Warm, kyu treatment using cones of moxa the size of a rice grain or smaller.

Chronic Fatigue Syndrome:
Inflammation of the nervous system; toxemia of the nervous system.

Chu Sho: Middle region of the abdomen. The starting point of the flow of meridian energy.

Congestion: Stagnation.

Danshin: Tapping the head of the needle with the thumbnail or index finger with a flicking motion. This technique helps address stuck needles.

Disease: An abnormality in Qi. Qi is either too weak or too strong. It occurs when congestion (stagnation) and toxemia (inflammation) exceed the capacity of the system to manage it.

Dojo: (place of the way) A hall or space for immersive learning or meditation attached initially to temples. It is considered a special place supported, managed, and cared for by the students, not the instructors. Traditionally, there is a front altar (Shomen) with a shrine (Kamidana) adorned with flowers, plants, and sculptures.

Eggplant: An edible nightshade plant used topically to "burn" warts off. The procedure involves taping the flesh of fresh, raw eggplant to the applicable site. Do not use the skin, just the interior "meat" of the plant. Cover the wart with the eggplant, tape it in place, and change it every four to eight hours until it disappears.

Empishin: Magnet/press tack.

Enhance: Replenish deficient Qi, what other schools call Ho.

Enshin: Non-inserted needle. It is less sharp than teishin.

Fu: (passage of contents) Of the hollow organs.

Fuki Shi-ge ike Ho: Taping around tsubo, causing vibration.

Fukushin: an abdominal diagnosis combined with kampo (herbal) treatment.

Goshin: Gold and silver needles.

Gyoshin: Fire needle.

GV #17: (Noko) The door of the brain.

Hara: A Japanese word that has no equivalent in English. It refers to the lower abdomen and the physical, spiritual, and metaphysical center of the human body.

Hari: (subtle needling) Needle therapy-style meridian therapy.

Many techniques are noninvasive. Hari therapy employs precise control and manipulation of Qi. Japanese-style acupuncture, in general, and meridian therapy use few needles and soft stimulation, hardly felt by the patient. Therefore, precise pulse diagnosis, point location, needling technique, and palpatory skills are of utmost importance. Striving throughout life to perfect these techniques is the mission – the goal.

Hibiki: Echo, noise, reverberation, sound. The presence of Qi transmits through the needle to the oshiate center of the practitioner's finger.

Hinaishin: Intradermal needling. Invented by Kobei Akabane. It is micro-acupuncture, small-dose therapy.

Ho: (enhance) Techniques to replenish Qi when depleted.

Honji-ho: (root treatment)

Treating the cause.

Hyoji-ho: (branch treatment) Relief of symptoms. Combining hon-ji and hyo-ji in go gyo meridian therapy is quite helpful.

Illustration of Acupuncture Points: Self- described as "basic information concerning the location of acupoint" and published by Ido-No-Nippon-Sha (1977 edition). It was my first commercially published meridian textbook.

Indo: On Tokumyaku between lower Tai Yo (Bl) #2, considered a unique Tai Yo point to treat sinus issues, lack of clarity.

Inflammation: Toxemia.

Inochi (Life) Medicine: An evolutionary perspective of traditional oriental rooted in Five Element meridian therapy and three yin/three yang diagnostics and therapeutics with a radical interpretation of the sun/kan/shaku pulses. Inochi (Life) Medicine became apparent through the study and practice of Kototama Life Medicine.

Jaku-Taku: A needling technique. After you plant the needle, manipulate it up and down, like a bird pecking, without removing it. Use a weak dose to stimulate the nervous system while sedating blood vessels and muscles; a significant dose for sedating the nervous system and simultaneously opening the blood vessels and relaxing muscles. What happens is within the ability of the practitioner.

Jingei-myaku-ko Pulse Diagnosis: A pulse diagnosis from about 300 CE to 1000 CE. Reintroduced in 1970 through the work of Dr. Doeki Oguro, jingei pulse diagnosis refers to a comparison of the carotid pulse at lower Yo Mei (St) #9 (jingei) with the radial pulse at upper Tai Yin (Lu) #9 (taien), sun position. Nakazono Osensei treated as sacred his new understanding of the Go Gyo (Five Elements) achieved through his 20-year journey that included the most in-depth studies of the Kototama Principle. The revelation of the jingei diagnosis demonstrates the harmonization of the Futonorito Five Element paradigm.

Furthermore, understanding the jingei diagnosis is how I came to realize the dominant arrangement of the roku-bu-jio-yi (wrist pulse diagnosis) is of another era and that there is another way to understand the wrist pulses.

Jitsu: Vital energy interrupted by disease related to Qi and Ketsu, resulting in excess. Jitsu condition will show on its junction point. If the pulse seems jitsu but does not indicate it on its junction point, it is not a jitsu condition; the kyo condition will not show out on this point.

Junetsu: Soft kneading muscle massage with a firm grip.

Kai-ShiBari: (taking back) Techniques to correct a mistake, such as errors in needling, forceful methods of treatment, using enhance/ho instead liberate/sha (and vice versa), or use of the wrong tsubo.

Kami- Spirit:

Ka – fire; male; heaven; vertical; time.

Mi - water; female; earth; horizontal; space.

Where ka meets mi [+] = Nakayima.

Kampo: Japanese traditional herbal medicine was advanced in the seventeenth century by Yoshimasu Todo, who developed a refined technique of abdominal palpation, <u>fukushin</u>, to provide additional information in determining the appropriate herbal formula.]

Kan San Ho: No needle; treat with tube only.

Kanjo (Kan): Position the middle finger on the wrist to take the pulse directly over the stylus process.

Kappo: (resuscitation method, restoration therapy). Techniques for physical body repair,

including tsubo treatment, tactile stimulation, physical manipulation, and alignment techniques.

Kei: Meridian.

Kei Ketsu: Main system.

Keiketsu: Regular meridian point.

Kei Ki: Extraordinary meridian.

Kei Myaku and Ryaku Myaku:

Main meridians and branches

(jing-Luo)/extraordinary meridian.

Kototama Institute: Opened in 1977 with Osensei conducting classes, leading Kototama sound practice and studies, and providing seminars and workshops. In

September 1978, he started a two-year training program in oriental medicine, acupuncture, and

Kototama Life Medicine; two years later, it became a three-year program.

Kototama Life Medicine: The guidance of universal energy, Qi, to facilitate the energetic equilibrium of body, spirit, and mind and show the expansion of human consciousness through attuning to the sound rhythms within spoken language. This universal energy, Qi, manifests the meridians and the vowel sounds: *A, I, E, O, U.* The universal energy expresses life-spirit *A* life-will, *I* Life-empowerment *E,* life-memory *O*, life-form *U.*

Kototama (Word Soul) Principle: Soul/spirit/power within the vocal sounds of human language through which reality is created and consciousness expressed. Sources are the *Kojiki* and *Takenouchi Documents*. Ueshiba Osensei, the founder of Aikido, introduced Nakazono Osensei to the sound principle. His pursuit of understanding led him to Ogasawara Sensei, whose lineage of Kototama studies traced to the nineteenth-century Meiji Restoration Period, and the family of calligraphers enlisted to translate the ancient scrolls known as the *Takenouchi Documents*.

Law and Therapy of Natural Medicine: Written and self-published for Nakazono Osensei students. The 1978 and 1979 editions, we called the "Red Book," the color of their covers. The 1980-1981 edition was the "Gold Book" for the same reason, plus being exceptionally rich in information.

Liberate: Disperse excessive Qi. What other schools call Sha.

Nan Jing: The Classic of Difficult Issues. Compiled around the first to second centuries of this era, it addresses issues relevant to the information in the *Neijing*, "Canon of Internal Medicine," also termed the "Yellow Emperor's Classic of Internal Medicine," compiled five hundred years earlier. *Nan Jing* presents the wrist pulses diagnosis.

Natural Life Therapy: Osensei studied consciousness and addressed words. He accepted responsibility for his spoken and penned words. He gave much thought and discussion to the naming of his system. To Sensei, it was Kototama Life Medicine, but he also sought a word sound that would be comfortable audibly and socially to the English-hearing brain, and he had some issues with the word "medicine." After much deliberation, he made peace with the term "Natural Life Therapy."

OA: MindSpirit - Intellectual expression of the spiritual dimension.

Ogasawara: Professor Koji Ogasawara of Tokyo, Japan, who founded Dai San Bummei Kai (the Third Civilization Association).

Oshiate: Since the seventeenth century, the technique of holding the needle with one hand while inserting it with the other, allowing for slight stimulation with very thin needles. It emphasizes locating tsubo by feeling the skin's surface with the fingers.

Pressure Pain: Watch face and body reactions. Severe, sharp pain is more significant than dull, achy pain. Do not cause too much discomfort to your patient. If there is no pain or discomfort in the abdomen, check from lower Yo Mei (St) #36 to lower Yo Mei (St) #38 and between the third and fourth toes. If pain or discomfort, provide teate.

Roku Bu Jio Yi: Both hands, six pulses; also termed sun-kan-shaku- bu-joi.

Ryaku: Vein or vessel.

Ryaku Myaku: Extraordinary meridians.

Saiki: Hari technique that guides and collects Qi at the needling point.

Sakai Hon Rei Teate: Hands healing spirit/spiritual handwork/spirit healing. Sakai Sensei termed his handwork teate ('hand- spirit-hand). He treated all conditions exclusively through the abdomen. Nakazono Osensei named it Sakai Hon Rei Teate, or Sakai's sacred way of healing through the hands. Teate assists the body in maintaining well-being and prevents the development of illness. We study teate for its health preservation as well as its healing power. With practice, the hands can enhance and liberate as skillfully as with hari.

San: Three.

San-Shin: Light rapid tapping of the surface skin without twirling the needle or purposefully piercing the skin.

Sansho: Triple heater, three burners, three spaces.

- Jo Sho: Upper Space - Located above the xiphoid process.
- Chu Sho: Middle Space - Between xiphoid process and navel
- Ka Sho: Lower Space - Below the navel

San In/San Yo:

Three Yin - Tai, Sho, Ketsu

Three Yang - Tai, Sho, Mei.

Sha (Liberate): Needling techniques to disperse excessive Qi.

Seikotsu-in: Traditional osteopathy techniques provided by judo masters in the late nineteenth century.

Sensei: Sen-before, sei- life; "one who proceeded you;" teacher.

Sesshoku: A hari treatment of making contact, light tapping on the skin without twirling the needle.

Shaketsu: Bloodletting.

Shaku-chu (Shaku): Space where the ring finger perceives the pulse. It is seven bu proximal to the kanjo (kan) position.

Shaku-ju:

- Shaku: Long-term accumulation of immobile stagnation of yin Qi.
- Ju: Current mobile stagnation of yang.

Shiatsu: Traditional Japanese physical manipulation by hand, finger, thumb, elbow, knee, and foot. It affects meridian energy to correct and maintain Qi, form, and function of the body and skeletal structure, joints, tendons, and muscles.

Shindo: (children of god) Children under seven years of age.

Shinsen: Vibration with the hand affects the peripheral nervous system and muscles.

Sho: Small, less. A place larger than mei.

Shonishin: Non-invasive pediatric acupuncture therapy.

Sotai: A system of simple movements devised by Keizo Hashimoto, MD, to restore and support a balanced posture and movement.

"So Wen": One of two sections of the *Nei Jing* (Yellow Emperor's Classic of Internal Medicine), titled "Classics of Dialogs Concerning Internal Medicine." The other part,

"Ling Shu," is a technical acupuncture instruction manual titled "Axis of the Divine Soul."

Stagnation: Congestion.

Successful Acupuncture Session: When the four steps of diagnosis, tsubo selection, needle insertion, and needle removal come together correctly. The most important is palpating the tsubo and inserting the needle, requiring many years of practice

Sugiyama's Three-Needle Principle:

1. Ju-atui: Manipulative therapy to pressure point.
2. Shiate: Pressure with the left hand
3. Shashite: Insertion with the right hand

Sunko (Sun): Position the index finger to read the pulse closest to the wrist. It is six bu from the kanjo position.

Tai: Great, large. Big, thick.

Tai Kyoku: (Chinese: Tai Chi) The void, supreme ultimate, center between heaven and earth.

Tai-Yo: Big Yang. The literal meaning is "sun."' Tai-Yo refers to the part of the body most exposed to sunlight; Yo-Mei is less exposed than Tai-Yo; Ketsu Yin is the most shielded part of the body. Tai Yin is less sheltered than Ketsu Yin; Sho Yin is the least protected. One herbal approach based on the Shokaron states that disease first spoils Tai Yo, Yo Mei, Sho Yo, Sho Yin, Tai Yo, and Ketsu Yin. (*Meridian Therapy, Part 2*; Fukushima Kodo; © 1991)

Takenouchi Documents: Ancient documents that have conscientiously recorded the history of humanity and Earth. The *Takenouchi Documents* were transcribed by Takenouchino Matori around 1,500 years ago from older texts in a mixture of Japanese and Chinese characters.

They were translated by Emperor Meiji's royal calligrapher, revealing the Kototama Principle.

Tanden: A specific area, physical and anatomical, of the abdomen and a physiological energetic space, which is the center. Located three tsun below the navel around Ninmyaku (CV) #5 (Sekimon) area. The place where Qi is intensive.

Taro root: Colocasia esculenta. It is a tropical, edible tuber plant used in Japanese folk medicine for drawing out fevers, infections, inflammations, and foreign objects; it reduces pain and accelerates the healing of fractures, blunt trauma, and some skin cancers.

Teate: Hand-healing-spirit. See Sakai Hon Rei Teate.

Teishin: A non-insertable needle that is sharper than enshin.

Tension: It may seem like a jitsu condition, but most seniors consider it a Kyo condition. A lack of tension is a good sign. No tension does not mean soft or loose muscles. Muscles that relax readily and allow stress to exist bilaterally are good signs.

"Three Civilizations" – The three consciousnesses, societies, and mentalities that are formed through the formulations of Sugaso, Kanagi, and Futonorito orders of language.

Toxemia: Inflammation.

Treatment Protocol: Go Gyo, SoSei, San Yin/San Yo. The emphasis is the pulse and abdominal diagnosis and natural care focusing on teate.

Tsubo: Acupuncture point. The source of the word is from pot, earthenware vessel, jar, or, more precisely, the nothingness of a jar. It is a vital point found in sensitivity. The name often speaks of its location, therapeutic effect, clinical significance, nature (yin/yang), and Go Gyo relationship. The connection between tsubo and meridians has more to do with functional than morphological and structural relationships. The phrase "hitting the tsubo" refers to something important being pinpointed ("hitting the nail on the head"). It is challenging to hit perfectly yet remarkably effective when done right. A responsible practitioner would never perform hari (needling) or okyu (moxibustion) on a tsubo (point) until palpated to find its precise location.

Tsun Measurement: (Use patient's fingers)
- 4 fingers = 3 sun
- 2 fingers = 1 ½ sun
- Width of pad = 1 sun

Yamaguchi Shido (1765-1842): Early explorer of Kototama Futomani. He taught Deguchi Onisaburo, who taught Morihei Ueshiba, who introduced Masahilo M. Nakazono to Kototama, *SU*.

Yang Kyo: Empty yang; unable to express or move.

Yang Reaction: An improvement in symptoms after treatment.

Yin Reaction: Nausea, vomiting, dull feeling, muscular/joint pain, lack of appetite, sleeplessness, additional symptoms appear, or current symptoms worsen following treatment. These symptoms usually dissipate in 24 hours.

Yin-Jitsu: Filled up, too much, over strong, concentrating activity resulting in an inability to receive.

Yin-Kyo means yin is void, weak, deficient, and unable to hold.

Yo: Yang.

Yo Mei: Yang bright.

Zo: Storing includes the liver, heart, spleen, lungs, kidneys, and heart constrictor.

Notes: